Diabetic Retinopathy for the Comprehensive Ophthalmologist

Jonathan D. Walker, M.D.

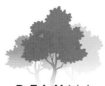

DELUMA
medicalpublishers

Lauren Fath Editing and Publishing
Chicago, IL

Deluma Medical Publishers
7900 West Jefferson Blvd.
Suite 300
Fort Wayne, IN 46804

Editor and Publisher:
Lauren Fath
879 N. Paulina St.
Chicago, IL 60622
847-903-9635
laurenfath@gmail.com

Layout and Design:
M. Walt Keys
182 Design
723 Park Ave.
Cincinnati, OH 45174
513-258-9635
walt@182design.com
www.182design.com

Line Art:
Roberta J. Sandy-Shadle
Publications
Indiana University-Purdue University, Fort Wayne

Legal Disclaimer

The author provides this material for educational purposes only. It is not intended to represent the only or best method or procedure in every case, nor to replace a physician's own judgment or give specific advice for case management. Including all indications, contraindications, side effects, and alternative agents for each drug or treatment is beyond the scope of this material. All information and recommendations should be verified, prior to use, with current information included in the manufacturers' package inserts or other independent sources, and considered in light of the patient's condition and history. Reference to certain drugs, instruments, and other products in this publication is made for illustrative purposes only and is not intended to constitute an endorsement of such. Some material may include information on applications that are not considered community standard, that reflect indications not included in approved FDA labeling, or that are approved for use only in restricted research settings. The FDA has stated that it is the responsibility of the physician to determine the FDA status of each drug or device he or she wishes to use, and to use them with appropriate patient consent in compliance with applicable law. The author specifically disclaims any and all liability for injury or other damages of any kind, from negligence or otherwise, for any and all claims that may arise from the use of, any recommendations or other information contained herein.

ISBN-13: 978-0-9821472-0-7

Dedicated to
Deborah, Lucius and Maria

ACKNOWLEDGEMENTS

There are many broad shoulders upon which this book stands. First of all, there are the pioneers of retinopathy treatment that have given us the tools that we have and the elegant studies that tell us how to use them. There are also the folks all around the world that are trying to provide even better therapies—they intuitively grasp the infinity of things not covered in Chapter 2. On a more personal level, I owe a great debt to all the attending physicians and ancillary staff at the Ohio State University, the USC/Doheny Eye Institute and the University of Iowa. They are not only busy performing all the tasks mentioned above; they also had to suffer through training me. Any bad advice found in this book, however, is something I made up and not something they taught me.

I want to thank Dr. Sandeep Nakhate, Dr. Robert Goulet III and Lucius Walker who were willing to spend their valuable time reviewing the first draft of the text and whose comments and suggestions were greatly appreciated. I particularly want to thank Dr. Alan "Patience is Your Most Valuable Surgical Tool" Kimura—whose intuitive grasp of all things retina is, and ever shall be, indispensible. Thanks also to Drs. Giorgio Dorin, David Sorg, Valerie Purvin, James Schmidt, Dale Fath and John Pajka who contributed to individual chapters in their respective specialties. Everyone's advice was invaluable and is reflected by anything in the book that is actually useful. Any errors that are still here exist solely because I either ignored their suggestions or because of subsequent misinterpretations of reality on my part.

Thanks to my editor and publisher, Lauren Fath, who had the yeoman's work of making the text readable and did the infinite number of things required to shepherd a book into your hands. Also thanks to M. Walt Keys, who did the layout and design and found all the cool images at the beginning of each chapter (the symbolism of which, given the new treatments we will soon have, should be obvious). Their creativity, energy and enthusiasm made assembling the book effortless and a true pleasure. (Their contact info is in the front matter if you have a book in you that is hankering to get out.)

The marvey line art was provided by Roberta Sandy-Shadle and the photos in Chapter 7 were done by James Whitcraft—both at Indiana-Purdue University, Fort Wayne. Mike Neeson of Iridex helped out by confirming my memories of lasers of old, and Larry Hubbard of the Wisconsin Reading Center generously shared his Zen Master knowledge of retinopathy grading.

Thanks to my partner—Matt Farber—who actually saw the patients while I was locked in my office Photoshopping laser spots, and thanks to my exemplary office staff for keeping everything going when I wasn't. Of course, there are no words to thank my wife and kids for doing all the real work while I alternately napped and typed on the couch. No soy nada sin ellos.

Finally, thanks to the referring doctors for entrusting me with their patients and especially thanks to the patients themselves, who extend the ultimate honor of entrusting us with their eyes.

TABLE OF CONTENTS

AN INTRODUCTION from the author

This book is designed to transfer useful skills for the clinical management of diabetic patients. It does not start with the fundamentals; instead, it is assumed that the reader has basic examination skills and is at least partially familiar with various tests, such as fluorescein angiography and optical coherence tomography.

Nor does this text offer an in-depth discussion of basic science or an exhaustive review of the available literature. Like the Basic and Clinical Science Course from the American Academy of Ophthalmology, there are some references given at the ends of most chapters for further information. However, if you want an in-depth look at the literature behind treating retinopathy, you are encouraged to review the sections on diabetes in any of the major ophthalmology texts, and in particular, Ryan's retina text. The American Academy of Ophthalmology's Focal Point from March 2003 on diabetic retinopathy by Drs. Fong and Ferris is also an excellent and succinct review.

Simply put, the goal of this book is to help make the trenches where most of us live a bit more comfortable.

The voice of this text is different from standard texts—something done in hopes of conveying useful information without too much tedium. However, as a wise person once said, "There is a fine line between clever and stupid." If anything offends or interferes with the smooth download of information, let me know.

Also, there are no absolutes here. Once you think you know the best way to do anything, you have lost the ability to learn. Try these suggestions and techniques, and if they don't work, throw them out. Run them by your mentors and your friendly neighborhood retinal specialists—get other opinions and synthesize a style of your own. I welcome any comments and/or complaints. If the gods of retina smile on this book, then perhaps there will be better editions with plenty of input from people way smarter than I am. My contact info is below.

Mostly, I hope that you can peruse these pages and find something that will help you to help patients who have one of the most prevalent and vicious causes of blindness on this planet.

Jonathan Walker, M.D.
Assistant Clinical Professor
Indiana University School of Medicine, Fort Wayne
Allen County Retinal Surgeons
7900 West Jefferson Blvd. #300
Fort Wayne, IN 46804
260 / 436.2181

P.S. At various points in the text, there are unavoidable opportunities to harass our surgical colleagues who have mastered more refractively oriented procedures. Recognize that this is meant in good sport and, in truth, stems largely from professional jealousy—they can actually understand things like high order aberrations and apodized lenses *and* they have patients who hug them after surgery.

Retina specialists do not generally get hugged by their patients. Moreover, the only bit of optics we understand is The Retina Refraction: room lights on—better one; room lights off—better two.

Onward…

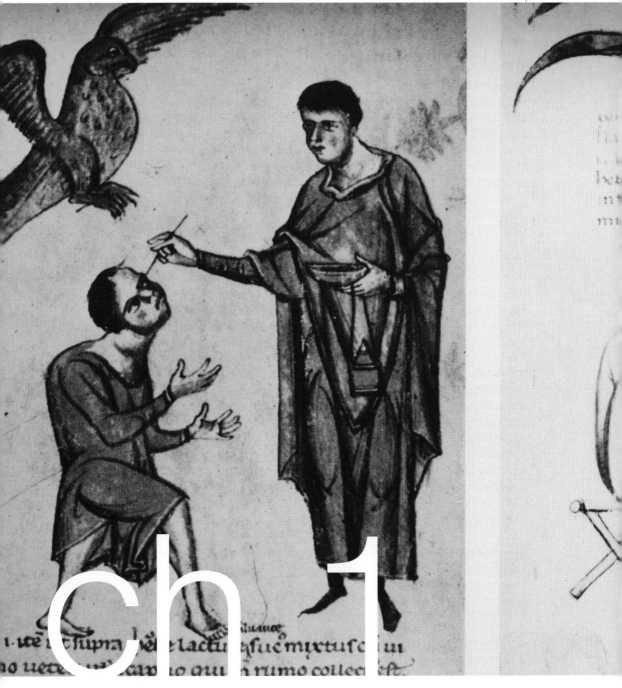

ch 1

A Tiny Bit of Statistics and a Big Pep Talk

First, some really big numbers: An estimated 20.2 million Americans have diabetes mellitus, and the number is expected to grow to over 30 million cases by the year 2025. Thanks to exports like the Great Western Lifestyle, the number of worldwide cases is expected to increase by 72%—to 333 million—by the year 2025. That is a lot of microaneurysms. By contrast, currently the number of patients blind from cataracts worldwide is estimated to be 18 million people. In other words, although a lot of ophthalmic effort is (correctly) directed towards decreasing the worldwide cataract burden, the number of patients at risk for vision loss from diabetes will soon be almost 20 times greater. Moreover, once a cataract is popped out, the job is done. Treating diabetes goes on forever for both the patient and physician—it ain't one-stop shopping.

Diabetic blindness also tends to occur at a time when people are younger and more active in society; it is the leading cause of new blindness in patients under the age of 65. The rate of onset is variable, but after 20 years, about 60% of Type 2 and essentially all Type 1 diabetics will have some sort of retinopathy. You will spend a great deal of time caring for these patients. It may seem that the treatment of diabetic retinopathy has been tremendously streamlined with the help of large clinical trials with which you are no doubt familiar. However, the reality is that each patient you see presents an incredibly complex array of variables—social, emotional, physical and retinal. Addressing all of these variables requires a lot more than the ability to memorize the definition of clinically significant macular edema. It is axiomatic that we all went into ophthalmology to avoid dealing with the morass of an entire patient. Unfortunately, when it comes to treating diabetic retinopathy, your results are going to suck if you don't start by understanding the entire patient. At the very least, recognize that by the time a diabetic needs your help, they are usually facing the risk of irreversible vision loss—real, life-changing, disabling vision loss—not Nerf vision loss that can be fixed with Lasik.

> **Dharma break:** Each diabetic patient whose vision you save probably represents more quality-of-life units than a whole surgery schedule full of 20/30 glare cataracts. Think about it…

And the battle is bigger than just honing your clinical skills and trying to deal with the entire patient. At the risk of sounding hyperbolic, you also have to look at the society in which you function. It has been said that if patients are examined in a timely fashion and the standard treatment guidelines are followed, less than 5% of diabetics will develop severe vision loss.[1] A huge part of your job lies in recognizing the importance of the first clause of that sentence: *if patients are examined in a timely fashion*. Not only do you need to develop the ability to treat these people, but you also have to be aggressive about getting them in to be seen. Far too many diabetics show up only when they start having symptoms, and this is just not the best way to keep people seeing.

Educate the patient and the patient's physicians at every visit. Educate the patient's family about the importance of getting everyone in the family routinely checked for diabetes and getting anyone who is diabetic in for an annual exam.

Educate society. Give talks at local diabetes support groups. Offer to provide information for the health desk editors at local newspapers, magazines or TV stations. Get involved with efforts to provide universal coverage. Do the free clinic thing. Make general information slides for the local cinema multiplex so they can be interspersed with all of those fascinating questions about which actor said what in which movie. Whatever. Just get these people in.

(All this may not only help prevent blindness; it can also help build your reputation and your practice—a twofer! Watch the ethical ramifications, though. It is one thing to generate public service messages that help patients and their doctors. It is quite another thing to plant your smiling face on an ad that says you are the bronzed god or goddess of retinopathy. This is a test…)

Unfortunately, a large part of your diabetic-treating career will consist of taking care of sad cases that didn't get in—hence the rationale for books like this. Helping a pair of eyes, and the patient attached to them, by slowing their descent into severe vision loss is still a good thing, but not a lot of fun. It is way better to body-slam the retinopathy before it can get to the fovea or up into the vitreous, but you can only do this if you see the patient before the real trouble begins. Aggressive monitoring and treatment can easily keep someone seeing until well after they leave the planet, which is something that you will hopefully be able to do many times and for many people before you hop off the globe, too.

References and Suggested Reading

1.   Rosenblatt B, Benson W. Diabetic Retinopathy. In: Yanoff M, Duker J, et al., editors. Ophthalmology, Second Edition. USA: Elsevier, 2004:877-886.

Wild S, Roglic G, Green A, Sicree R, King H. Global prevalence of diabetes: estimates for the year 2000 and projections for 2030. Diabetes Care 2004;27:1047-53.

Zhang X, Norris SL, Saadine J, et al. Effectiveness of interventions to promote screening for diabetic retinopathy. Am J Prev Med 2007;33:318-35.

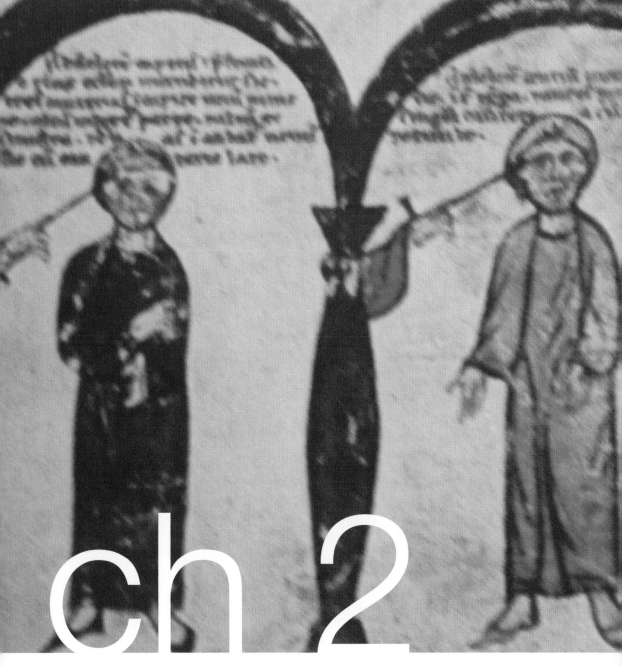

ch 2

Basic Science

BASIC SCIENCE

Didn't you read the intro? This is not a basic science text. If you want basic science, get a real textbook. Or go to ARVO. Sheesh...

moving on >>

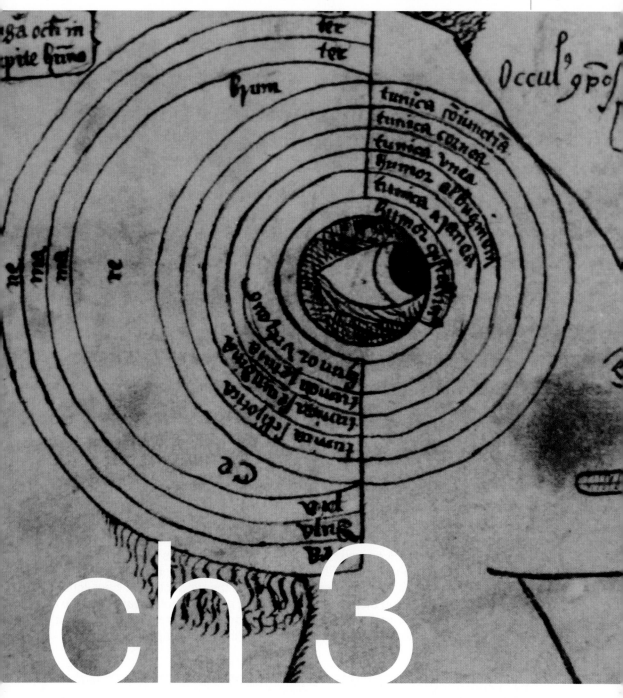

ch3

Know Your Weapons—Lasers and Their Ilk

PART A. Laser Physics for Wimps

This section really does not have a heck of a lot to do with patient care issues, but it is useful to have some idea about how the little demons inside the laser box do their thing. First of all, it is impossible to talk about lasers without rehashing the acronym. At some point in your career you may come across a pedant that uses your ability to regurgitate the meaning of "LASER" in order to determine whether you are a worthwhile physician. So never forget that laser stands for Light Amplification by Stimulated Emission of Radiation. But what does that mean?

The fundamental thing to remember is that the electrons orbiting the atomic nucleus want to ditch their extra energy and get to lower levels. This process results in the emission of photons.

It turns out that electrons can release photons of only certain wavelengths because electrons can only live in certain orbitals, which are determined by the atom in which the electron resides. If the electron falls to a lower orbit, the electron releases a photon whose energy corresponds exactly to the difference in energy between the two orbitals—no in-betweenies allowed. The electron can also be bumped up to a higher orbital if it happens to absorb a photon of the exact energy that matches the energy difference between the lower and upper orbitals. If you can bump a bunch of electrons up to a given orbital and then get them to drop back down to a lower level at the same time, you can—for instance—stop diabetic retinopathy.

Getting the electrons to do this involves a weird and mysterious variation of the whole bumping up and dropping down process (this is where the Stimulated Emission part comes from). It turns out that if a photon happens to have the same energy as the difference between the pumped-up orbit where an electron is and the next-lowest orbit, and if said photon happens to pass by one of these electrons—without hitting it—the photon will stimulate the electron to drop into the lower orbit and produce a second photon that is coherent (meaning the peaks and troughs of the waves of both photons occur at the same time). It is this rather amazing property that allows the production of laser light from a host of stimulated electrons. Furthermore, a given photon can stimulate a whole bunch of electrons as it whizzes by, and each photon released will go out and stimulate the release of even more photons (the Light Amplification part of LASER).

> **In 1917,** Albert discovered that the oscillating field of the stimulating photon perturbs the electron's field, which causes it drop to the lower energy level sooner than it otherwise would. It took several decades, however, to turn this theoretical knowledge into something that even an ophthalmologist could use.

Older lasers use some type of gas to provide a population of high-energy electrons for this process to occur. You can usually identify a gas ion laser because it tends to be large with big black cables running from the laser to the wall; many such lasers are also water cooled, which adds a gurgling-broken-toilet ambience to the treatment experience. The gas molecules are "pumped" by either an electric discharge or a powerful light source, which creates a large population of high-energy electrons. There is also a fully reflective mirror at one end of the gas tube and a partially reflective mirror at the other. This makes the photons bounce back and forth a bit, which ensures that as many electrons as possible are stimulated to drop to a lower orbit and release a photon. Only a small amount of photons escape through the partially reflective mirror and this, in turn, produces the laser light that you then put into a patient's eye.

Nowadays, most lasers generate coherent light from a light emitting diode; such lasers tend to be much smaller and look not unlike a home theatre amp, but with fewer buttons. These diode, or solid-state, lasers are a bit more complicated to explain. They involve things such as electrons moving from high-energy conduction bands to low-energy valence bands, skipping altogether the delightfully named "forbidden region" of energy. This sets up a situation where stimulated emission can occur in a chunk of matter that is much smaller than the gas tube of an older laser. Electrical energy is used to shove electrons into the higher valence levels and the release of photons is stimulated at the junction of the diode. The diode itself is still sandwiched between mirrors, just like in a gas tube laser. The whole process is far more efficient than in a gas laser, hence the lack of big cables and pipes which made gas ion lasers unsuitable for use as laser pointers.

Lasers used to treat retinal diseases are known as continuous wave lasers because the laser beam can be generated, well, continuously. The user sets the actual duration of the beam, and the power output is relatively low, which allows a gradual, controlled response in the target tissue. This is in contrast to the "pulse lasers" that are used in ophthalmology—the neodymium: yttrium-aluminum-garnet laser (Nd: YAG) and the excited dimer laser (excimer). This type of laser puts all of its energy output into a very brief period of time. Because the energy is the power per unit of time, a laser pulse released in a very short time can have a very high peak power, which, if focused in a small spot, can reach an extremely high power density (irradiance) and can essentially be explosive.

The frequency of light generated by a laser depends on the substance being used to generate the light. If the frequency produced is not ideal for the chosen application, it can be changed by using either harmonic generation or organic dyes. An organic dye laser can produce a spectrum of wavelengths, but such lasers are inefficient—a lot of energy is lost when the primary laser is fired into the dye to excite and lase its fluorescence spectrum in the dye laser cavity. Dye lasers tend to be expensive and difficult to maintain, and you are not likely to see such a laser nowadays.

Harmonic generation is a far more common technique for changing a laser's frequency. In this case, the laser light is passed through a special crystal that will vibrate at the laser's frequency and generate harmonics that are multiples of the laser's frequency. Such crystals are commonly used to double the frequency of the output of a YAG laser in order to produce a wavelength in the green spectrum (i.e., from 1064 to 532 nm). A typical diode green laser generates light in this fashion.

All of this is a horribly oversimplified explanation of one of the mainstays of retinal therapy. If you ever want to feel overwhelmed, pick up a bona fide textbook on lasers to get an idea of how complex they really are. Ultimately, we all have to be very grateful for the fact that there are plenty of good folks out there that actually understand this stuff on a fundamental level and are always working to give us better and better tools. This way we can concentrate on part B.

PART B. From Acronym to Verb: Lasering People

Once you manage to get your hands on a laser and point it at a patient, you can expect three types of tissue interactions, depending on the nature of the laser: photocoagulation, photodisruption and photoablation. These categories are a bit arbitrary because they are really part of a spectrum of how tissues respond to laser energy. It is convenient, though, to use these terms to distinguish the tissue effects of the different types of ophthalmic lasers. For instance, if you devote your life to fighting the demon scourge known as spectacles, you will depend on photoablation to provide your worldly needs. In this case, an excimer laser generates a wavelength of 193 nm (in the ultraviolet range), which can break chemical bonds. This allows very precise removal of tissue with only minimal damage to the surrounding structures. Photoablation is definitely a "now you see it, now you don't" kind of thing.

When you perform a YAG peripheral iridectomy or capsulotomy, you will be depending on photodisruption. This is more of a mechanical effect that results from tightly focused, high-power laser light, which produces an explosively expanding vapor bubble of ionized plasma. This bubble then quickly collapses, producing acoustic shockwaves that happily blow apart the structure you are treating. This is very satisfying from a single-player-shooter point of view, but it is not particularly user-friendly when you want to treat something delicate and squishy like the retina.

Retinal laser treatment depends on the far more gentlemanly tissue effect known as photocoagulation. In this case, the laser literally cooks the tissue at a microscopic level. The resulting coagulation of proteins causes the desired effect — hopefully without any photoablative or photodisruptive pyrotechnics.

> **There is a fourth tissue interaction** — photochemical — but you are unlikely to use it. In this case, a very low-power laser is used to activate a specific chemical to obtain the desired effect in the tissue. The use of a red laser to activate verteporfin (Visudyne) in order to treat neovascular age-related macular degeneration is the best example of this.

PART C. The Most Important Stuff

Regardless of how the laser is produced, there are certain variables that you need to intuitively understand if you are going to treat patients safely and effectively. The first one is the wavelength of the laser you use. Figure 1 is the classic display of how each laser color is absorbed in various ocular tissues. For a long time, people hoped that different colors would allow one to customize the treatment depending on the indication. For instance, you can see that yellow really nails one of the peaks of oxyhemoglobin relative to green, and if you ever have occasion to use a yellow laser, you can detect a significant difference in how, for instance, microaneurysms respond to a different wavelength (they tend to be very easy to pick off with the yellow—often with very little disruption of the retinal pigment epithelium and outer retina).

Perhaps more clinically significant is both the marked dropoff in hemoglobin absorption and the gradual dropoff in melanin uptake as you move into the red end of the spectrum. This explains in part why red and infrared burns require more power and tend to penetrate deeper into the more pigmented choroid. It also helps explain why the infrared diode laser in particular is so different to use relative to a green laser.

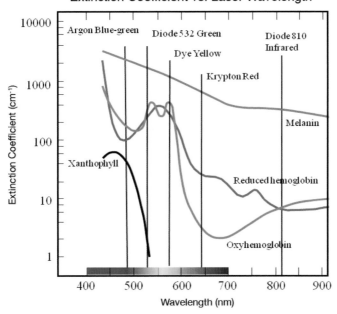

Figure 1. The absorption of different laser wavelengths by different substances in the retina, RPE and choroid. Note that, in general, the further you go toward red, the less the absorption—hence the need for more power and a resultant deeper burn with longer wavelengths. You can also see how yellow hits a peak of oxyhemoglobin absorption relative to green, which accounts for the difference in how microaneurysms are affected by each wavelength. Finally, you can see why it is a very bad idea to use blue light anywhere near the fovea, where xanthophyll pigment is found. (Data from Mainster MA. Wavelength selection in macular photocoagulation. Tissue optics, thermal effects, and laser systems. Ophthalmology 1986;93:952-8.)

However, although one does get different tissue responses depending on the wavelength, no one has proven that there is a huge difference in the ultimate treatment effect. Besides, you will basically be using whatever laser has been plopped in your clinic because there is no way you can go out and shop and compare with these enormously expensive devices. Fortunately, most of the studies on diabetic retinopathy were performed using some sort of green wavelength—usually argon green or its kissin' cousin diode green—and that is pretty much the standard color of laser found anywhere. Some places do have the fancy lasers that can generate different colors, and you should experiment with these colors for yourself. (Plus, there are few things cooler than the appearance of yellow or orange light coming from an ophthalmic laser.) Because multicolor lasers are as rare as Bugattis, though, the rest of this book will assume you have some sort of green laser to work with. Go Irish.

> **You may read references to "argon blue-green."** This is because 488 and 514 nm wavelengths were simultaneously available on older argon lasers. The 488 nm blue wavelength became déclassé and was eliminated because of increased uptake by xanthophyll pigment in the fovea and an increased risk of causing burns in yellowish nuclear sclerotic cataracts. (Look at the uptake of xanthophyll in Figure 1—this is not a subtle effect.) If you have an argon laser that actually has both lines don't ever use it for treating the retina, unless the blue line has been properly suppressed. You might be able to sell it on eBay as an antique, though. Ask your chairman first.

The one thing to remember for sure with any wavelength is what you learned in second-grade science class: Black absorbs everything and white reflects everything. In other words, if you are treating happily in an area of the retina and you come upon a dark area like a nevus or a previous laser scar, you need to watch out, because you can get an explosive burn as the pigment sucks in the laser (higher absorption translates in higher photothermal elevation). Remember to Turn It Down When You Hit Brown (and Cut Way Back When You Hit Black). Alternatively, if you need to treat a very pale area, you will need to crank it up—but be super careful when you hit pigment again.

FLUENCE

Although wavelength is fun to theorize about, the power density, or irradiance, and the energy density, or fluence, of the laser beam are the most important concepts to master if you are going to be a safe and effective laserist. Here, for completeness, are the only formulas in the book:

$$\text{Irradiance (W/cm}^2) = \frac{\text{Power (Watts)}}{\text{Spot Area (cm}^2)}$$

$$\text{Energy (Joules)} = \text{Power (Watts)} \times \text{Time (Seconds)}$$

$$\text{Fluence (J/cm}^2) = \frac{\text{Power (Watts)} \times \text{Time (Seconds)}}{\text{Spot Area (cm}^2)} = \frac{\text{Energy (Joules)}}{\text{Spot Area (cm}^2)}$$

We will try to stay away from the obligatory discussion of energy, work, radio-metric terminology, etc. that often shows up at this point in real textbooks. The key thing is that your laser output has a certain level of mojo and you need to know exactly how to control it.

Look at the last equation for fluence. Note that going up or down on power (Watts) or on exposure duration (time) creates a linear increase or decrease in the energy delivered. This means that if you are getting a good burn and you de-cide to, say, double the exposure duration, then you *have* to decrease the power or you will really cook things. It is hard to imagine why on earth one would want to do this when one is getting a good burn, but this is always mentioned in basic laser texts and it does help ensure that you understand the relationship. The really significant thing is that the clinical effect tends to be very intuitive—a mild increase in the power or duration will give you a mild increase in your burn, and the same is true if you want to turn things down.

However, because we are dealing with a biological system and not a photom-eter, it turns out that the relationship between the energy delivered and the type of burn that you get is a bit more complex. The exact same energy can result in different burns because the burn depends on how the laser is absorbed and how the heat is transmitted by the tissue. In other words, fiddling with the laser power and duration *generally* results in a common-sense change in the degree of uptake—a little more time or power results in a little more burn and a lot more time or power results in a lot more burn. But don't depend on this absolutely. Let's take another colorful box break.

> **Colorful Box Break:** Since you are basically using your laser to warm up the retina, you do need to be careful about using high powers at short dura-tion, because the nice linear relationship breaks down and you can end up microwaving the proverbial poodle of urban legend.* Your "typical" laser burn is determined not only by the energy density but also by the rate of heat transfer out of the burn area. Unfortunately, heat transfer is governed by factors far more complicated than the weenie-pre-med-physics equation above. For instance, heat transfer explains why it is easy to get a burn in the retina but really hard to get a burn on a big blood vessel—the blood "carries" away the heat and you can't get the vessel wall to cook easily. Because you should treat a big vessel exactly never, the real point of all this is that if you use a lot of power over a really short duration, there is not time for the heat to spread out and you can get a much hotter burn than you would expect if the response of the tissue were truly linear. To repeat: Stuffing a lot of power into a short duration can become explosive—you are going from a slow cook to a fast boil. This will be important in the next paragraph…
>
> (*Yes, this is a sophomoric metaphor, but if sleazy skull imagery will help you remember this point it is worth it.)

THE EFFECT OF SPOT SIZE

Going back to the mini-equations above, note that the irradiance (or power density) and the fluence (or energy density) are an inverse function of the *square* of the spot size—i.e., a small change in spot size can make a big difference in the irradiance and in the fluence you pour into the retina if you don't compensate by changing the power or duration. With a lot of energy delivered into a small spot, you can create a "YAG effect" because you will raise the temperature so fast and so high that the water in the tissue will actually boil. This is especially likely if you are also using a brief duration (less time for heat transfer, remember). The result is an explosively expanding bubble of water vapor that will cause a hole or hemorrhage or both. (Technically, it won't be a true YAG photodisruptive effect—there won't be any plasma formation—but the explosive vaporization of water in the tissue will have the same destructive physical effect, complete with a sickening pop-like sound in the patient's head. You can really mess up an eye doing this—and lose lots of style points with your patients and colleagues. We will return to this concept several times in this book to be sure it sinks in—it has to be internalized to your lizard brain parts just like the mental switch that keeps you from engaging phaco when you are next to the posterior capsule.)

Anyway, if you make the spot size smaller—even if it is only a little bit smaller—you really have to be religious about decreasing the other parameters so that you don't start punching holes in the retina. For instance, you might be using a strong power to cut through media opacities and you might also be using a short duration to try to make the laser less painful for the patient (no worries—much more on these techniques later). You might then decide to decrease the spot size in order to get an even better burn—a smaller spot will not spread out as much as a large spot if the view is hazy. If you do this, then you must cut back on power and work your way back up to a safe burn; otherwise, you will have increased irradiance and fluence by the square of the difference in spot size, and you will very likely cause a dangerously hot burn. Repeat: You *must* cut back on power and work your way back up to a safe burn if you decrease the spot size.

Also, remember that your spot size is not exclusively dependent on the setting you put on the slit lamp adapter. As we will see next chapter, each type of contact lens will minify or magnify the size of the actual spot projected on the retina. If you switch to a different contact lens, you might be shrinking the actual spot size without realizing it—thus dramatically changing how much power is focused onto the retina.

There are even more ways the spot size can change unintentionally. When you are working in the retinal periphery, your spot will sometimes shrink down as you treat through the edge of the patient's lens. Or if you are doing a macular laser in an area of swollen retina, the thickened retina will tend to diffuse the beam, and when you move to an area of thin retina, your spot effectively shrinks. Or when you are starting your laser career, it may take way longer than you want to get anything into focus and you may decide to fire away before your focus is crisp because you are frustrated. If the gods of retina then suddenly put your aiming beam into perfect focus, your spot will shrink down and suddenly you will be burning holes in important parts of your patient. Again, all this will be covered in greater detail in upcoming chapters—but the point is that your spot size may change whether you want it to or not, and you have to be ready to anticipate these changes and alter your parameters accordingly.

> **There is yet another way** that the biology of lasering can get you into trouble even without using small spots, and this occurs when you are using powers, for whatever reason, that are causing very hot burns. In this case, the very center of the spot can get hotter than the periphery. Heat building up in the periphery of the burn can at least dissipate into untreated retina, but heat building up in the center of the burn is trapped and cannot spread out much. The result is a sudden hemorrhage at the center of the burn if the uptake increases even a little bit (such as when going into more pigmented areas). As will be discussed in upcoming chapters, it is unlikely that you would be trying to create such a hot burn to treat diabetic retinopathy. It is important to know all the ways that things can go bad, though.

Time for a Paragraph That Begins With the Phrase "The Bottom Line…"

The bottom line is that you will have three variables that you can control from the front panel of your laser and slit lamp adapter. The power and the duration are mostly linear and tend to be fairly forgiving if you make small adjustments at a time. Spot size, however, is the one variable that is truly exponential and you have to keep this in mind if you are switching to smaller spots. You must turn down the power and titrate back up. By the way, it may seem daunting when the process of lasering a retina is "unpacked" into all these component parts. One gets a sense that it will take about 30 minutes to line up each shot after tinkering with power, duration and spot size. Actually, there are many tricks to controlling these variables quickly and effortlessly and, well, you are just going to have to read the rest of the book to find out.

> **OK.** Suppose all of these variables seem too confusing. Let's get basic and remember what a burn is. The retina is normally a beautifully transparent structure. If the organization of the proteins and cells is disrupted then it begins to lose its transparency, in the same way the cornea begins to become cloudy when it swells. A mild burn means that, literally, the retinal proteins are gently cooked so that the retina becomes translucent—it gets a slight grayish color as light begins to be mildly scattered. You can still see choroidal details through a light gray burn. As the burn gets hotter there is more disruption of the protein matrix and there is more scattering of light and the retina gets whiter and whiter—the choroidal detail is masked by the opaque white retina. If you are treating a patient and suddenly your burns get very white, please stop immediately and adjust your settings—the easiest thing to do is turn down the power—so that you do not start blowing holes in things.

MISCELLANEOUS Odds & Ends

Lasering in the Infrared

Infrared diode lasers tend to be cheaper and relatively bulletproof (their design is simpler than a frequency-doubled green diode laser and they require way less fuss than a gas laser). If cost or logistical considerations are important, you may have no choice but to use infrared. This could be problematic because infrared is much trickier to use. Appendix I talks a bit about the special needs of learning this wavelength—best to carve through the basic techniques covered in this book, and then you can read the stuff in the appendix to get ready to use infrared.

Micropulse and Other "No Touch" Lasers

There are lots of wondrous things to be found in the halls of diabetic retinopathy treatment. This might be one of them. Not a common technique, micropulse laser involves delivering only a fraction of the requested power over the duration of a burn. It does this by delivering laser energy in pulses rather than continuously, and it brings into the mix a cool new term: duty cycle. This is simply the percentage of time that the pulses are actually delivering laser power relative to the total time of the exposure (Figures 2 and 3). The pulsing keeps the temperature from building up in the same way it would with a continuous wave and allows a gentle subclinical effect without the creation of a visibly identifiable burn.

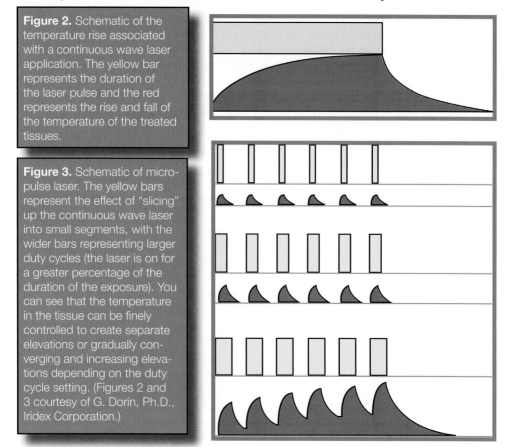

Figure 2. Schematic of the temperature rise associated with a continuous wave laser application. The yellow bar represents the duration of the laser pulse and the red represents the rise and fall of the temperature of the treated tissues.

Figure 3. Schematic of micropulse laser. The yellow bars represent the effect of "slicing" up the continuous wave laser into small segments, with the wider bars representing larger duty cycles (the laser is on for a greater percentage of the duration of the exposure). You can see that the temperature in the tissue can be finely controlled to create separate elevations or gradually converging and increasing elevations depending on the duty cycle setting. (Figures 2 and 3 courtesy of G. Dorin, Ph.D., Iridex Corporation.)

This approach is felt to create a very localized treatment effect—for instance, warming only the retinal pigment epithelium without affecting the underlying choroid or overlying retina.

How does it work? Well, since no one knows how any retinal laser really works, it is hard to say, but the philosophy would be that if a gnarly scar gets the job done, then perhaps gently heating cells without disrupting them might have some effect without necessarily causing permanent damage. There is a small literature suggesting that this approach can be effective, but at this point in time it is not clear how such techniques fit into the armamentarium—there are no large-scale controlled trials. There are other laser techniques being evaluated that are similar in philosophy—they all try to create a clinical effect without a destructive visible burn. The ultimate goal would be to use such techniques, perhaps in combination with pharmacologic treatments, in order to treat retinopathy without causing irreversible structural changes in the retina. It is worth keeping an eye on all these approaches—and if future studies demonstrate clear-cut efficacy, you can use this book for kindling or compost…

References and Suggested Reading

L'Esperance FA. Ophthalmic lasers, 3rd ed. St. Louis: Mosby, 1989.

Folk JC, Pulido JS. Laser photocoagulation of the retina and choroid. San Francisco: American Academy of Ophthalmology, 1997.

Singerman LJ, Coscas GJ. Current techniques in ophthalmic laser surgery, 3rd ed. Boston: Butterworth-Heineman, 1999.

Luttrull JK, Musch DC, Mainster MA. Subthreshold diode micropulse photocoagulation for the treatment of clinically significant diabetic macular oedema. Br J Ophthalmol 2005;89:74-80.

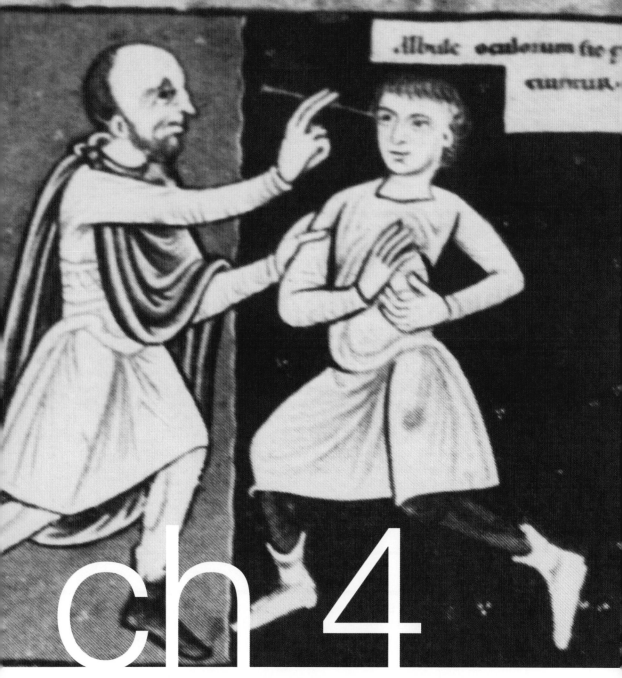

ch 4
Contact Lenses and the Wrangling Thereof

Becoming familiar with the contact lenses that are used to treat diabetic retinopathy is crucial. It is assumed that you have already mastered typical indirect non-contact lenses, such as the 90-diopter lens. But it turns out that contact lenses require a very different skill set, so they get their own chapter.

Contact lenses come in two main types: direct view lenses, such as the Goldmann three mirror, and inverted image lens system such as the Rodenstock. But first, a brief editorial…

This chapter will refer to several types of lenses. If you look at the manufacturers' catalogs, you will see that there are zillions of options. How can you try them to see whether they work for you? One option is to go to the manufacturers' exhibits at conventions. You will get a chance to try them all, but they never work as well on patients as they do on the little model eyes they use to demonstrate the lenses.

Another option is to dig around the back of all the drawers where your laser is kept. You will likely find a host of abandoned lenses, especially if you are in a large group practice or academic setting. Sometimes you will quickly realize why a given lens is in the graveyard, but sometimes you will find a real friend that works great for you. This also saves you a trip to the Academy meeting.

Above all, do not be fooled by the advertising that will have you thinking you will be able to treat patients effortlessly if you buy just the right lens. As you begin grappling with contact lenses, it is easy to think that your problems are due to the lens and that, somewhere over the rainbow, there is a perfect lens that will solve all your problems. You need to get over this phase quickly (otherwise, you will be spending a lot of money on lenses). It just takes practice— there is no secret magic lens.

Point-Counterpoint Box so the Lens Manufacturers Don't Get Too Ticked-off by the Previous Box Because We Need and Appreciate Their Constant Innovations

Although there is no magic lens that gets you over the hump of the learning curve, there is something to be said for having lenses that differ in subtle ways in order to address different nuances of treatment. Just like some guitarists prefer having a bunch of different instruments and others always use one favorite axe, you may find that you do better with lots of different lenses, or you may be happy with only one or two. Ultimately, this is something you will decide on your own once you have some skills with the basic lenses, so read on.

DIRECT VIEW LENSES

The direct view lenses are the easiest and most intuitive to use. The archetype is the Goldmann three mirror lens. This is the lens to have if you are stranded on your basic desert island, because it can do everything reasonably well. The direct (non-inverted) nature of the view means that once you get the lens on the patient, you are simply looking in a straight line through the pupil to the area of interest. The various mirrors then allow you to visualize segments of the periphery. Some Goldmann lenses have a small flange that fits behind the lids and helps to keep the lens in the patient's eye; it is a good idea to take advantage of such a flange when you are learning, because it is harder for the patient to blink the lens out once you get it in the eye. (More specific tips on actually getting the lens where you want it to go are covered in Chapter 7.)

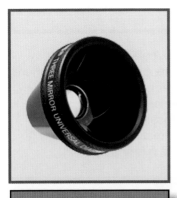

Figure 1. A typical three mirror Goldmann lens. (Courtesy of Ocular Instruments.)

The mirrors are set at different angles, with most Goldmann-type lenses having one mirror for the anterior chamber angle and two mirrors for different latitudes of the fundus. There are, however, variations on the Goldmann which have multiple mirrors at slightly different angles to get better coverage of the retinal periphery (the Karickhoff lens, for instance, has four mirrors).

The direct view makes it relatively easy to line up the lens so you can see the posterior pole, and you do not need to invoke the mental gymnastics that are necessary to use lenses that have an inverted image. Unfortunately, the field of view is rather small compared to the indirect lenses, and you will be more dependent on the patient's cooperation if you need to get to different areas. Also, direct lenses need a widely dilated pupil, and media opacities can be a real pain, because you cannot work around them as you can with an inverting lens.

Because the mirrors are set at a fixed angle and there is a small field of view, you need to make sure that you do not miss areas that lie between the latitudes most easily seen in each mirror. If you cannot quite get the view you need because the place you want to see is just outside the limited view provided by the mirrors or the direct view to the posterior pole, you do have some options. You can rock the lens back and forth to get more anterior and posterior exposure as you are treating the retina. The patient can also help you by looking a bit away and toward the mirror to accomplish the same goal. Finally, you can also use the contact lens as a gentle lever to push the eye in different directions. This last option can be done with any type of contact lens, and it is an important skill that will give you a lot of control over the eye. For instance, if the patient has had a retrobulbar block, you have to use the lens to move the eye around to see different areas. You also need to maintain the proper alignment when you do this, though, because if you angle the lens too much as you push the eye in different directions, you will lose your view. You have to fine-tune your finger proprioception so that you automatically know how the lens is oriented as you move it in different directions. (Figure 8 will elaborate on this.)

> **Important safety tip:** If the eye has not been blocked and you are pushing with your lens in order to move it around, you may inadvertently demonstrate the oculo-cardiac reflex—especially if you happen to be treating a patient who is nervous and uncomfortable (and this goes double if they are young males—triple if they have Harley-Davidson tats). Always remind a patient who is about to get their first laser to let you know if they begin to feel light-headed or dizzy, and if they do, stop the laser immediately and have them do the head-between-the-knees thing or even lie down on the floor. For some patients, the time between this light-headed sensation and becoming unconscious is rather short, and you lose many points with the family if your patient's face finds the cross members of the slit lamp table on its way to the ground. This concept is important enough that it is repeated at various points around the book.

Because you cannot get a very big picture with the "keyhole" view through the pupil, you also need to be very careful that your treatment is not extending more posteriorly than you wish. This can occur with the larger mirror and is especially likely if you are working temporally, where there are no large blood vessels to warn you that you are crossing into the macula. It is possible to inadvertently angle the lens and treat into the posterior pole without realizing it, especially if the patient happens to be looking in the direction of the mirror (Figure 2).

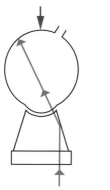 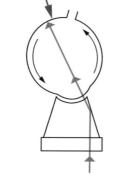

Figure 2. If you are using a Goldmann three mirror, you have to be very careful about where you are treating with the large mirror. It is possible to accidentally get well into the posterior pole, especially if the patient is looking toward the mirror. The red arrow represents the fovea as it moves toward the line of treatment when the eye rotates toward the mirror.

There is another type of direct view lens that is designed exclusively for viewing the posterior pole. In some institutions these lenses are referred to as pancake lenses, presumably because they're smaller than a Goldmann three mirror and because they do not have mirrors (perhaps these qualities make ophthalmologists think of pancakes). An example of this is the Yanuzzi lens, although there are many other types that are available.

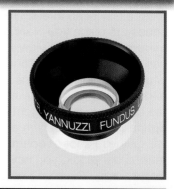

Figure 3. Yanuzzi macular contact lens. Note the very wide flange. This can take a bit of work to get into the eye, but it really locks the lens onto the eye once it is behind the lids. (Courtesy of Ocular Instruments.)

These lenses often have a very large flange that really keeps the lens behind the eyelids—you may even be able to let go of the lens so the patient can sit back and rest and it will remain in place. Although the overall field of view is limited by the direct line of sight, and these lenses are more dependent on patient cooperation, they give a breathtaking sense of the thickness of the retina. You should try to use them as much as possible, especially as you are learning the trade. The axial magnification and clarity of these lenses can really help you comprehend the nature of diabetic macular edema and help you get a feel for the three-dimensional location of the pathology. The patient's retina becomes a wonderland as you gleefully pluck microaneurysms from perches that suddenly seem yards above the underlying RPE. After you have a few exams under your belt with one of these lenses, you will understand what diabetic macular edema is about in a way that no ocular coherence tomography scan can capture. You will also appreciate what a feeble imitation of reality you get when you use a 90- or 78-diopter lens—no matter what the advertisements say. However, studying a lot of patients with a macular lens like this will enable you to be a much more effective examiner when you decide to cut corners and use a 90 or 78.

By the way, there are some other options to try to get a nice stereoscopic view without resorting to a contact lens—but like most things in life, the easier way is usually not the best way. You can get a 60-diopter lens (or something close to that number). The lower dioptric power will give you more axial magnification— you will get an enhanced stereoscopic view that can be almost as good as a contact lens. However, it is harder to line up both of your eyes through a 60-diopter; the patient has to be very well dilated and cooperative. If you can easily get the info you need from such a lens, then more power to you, but usually it is better to just put on the contact lens.

Another non-contact option is the Hruby lens. This is a plano-concave gizmo that can be attached to the front of your slit lamp. It works by neutralizing the corneal curvature from a distance, and you usually click it down or lift it into a slot so that it is directly in your line of sight, and then you can study a non-inverted image of the macula. There is only a small field of view, and you are very dependent on patient cooperation, but the stereo is pretty good. Most folks find that the Hruby is too tricky to use, but you should at least try it if you have one on your slit lamp.

INDIRECT LENSES

The indirect lenses will give you an excellent field of view compared to direct view lenses, but they require more finesse to obtain said field of view. An example of this type of lens would be the various Mainster lenses made by Ocular Instruments or the classic—but no longer manufactured—Rodenstock Panfundoscope (Figure 4). Volk also makes a selection of indirect lenses (Figures 5 and 6). All of these lenses essentially do the same thing that your 90-diopter lens does, but they are stuck to the eye to hold the eyelids open (and they throw in a few more optical elements to kick up the view a notch). You get an inverted image that, once you master the technique, allows you to treat a large area with minimal dependence on the patient's ability to cooperate.

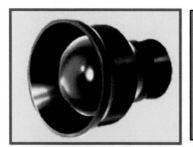

Figure 4. The Rodenstock Panfundoscope. This is a classic lens with an even more classic name. The design is handy because it is long, rather than wide, so it can get under Cro-Magnon brows and the length allows a lot of leverage for torquing the eye. Unfortunately, it is no longer manufactured. Volk makes a substitute, but the newer lens is smaller and works somewhat differently.

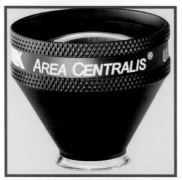

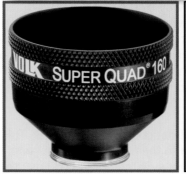

Figure 5. This is a more typical contemporary wide-field indirect contact lens. It is much shorter than the Rodenstock and can be a tight fit into a recessed eye, but the field of view does tend to be better. (Courtesy of Volk Optical.)

Figure 6. A typical indirect contact lens for macular treatment. Note the more subtle flange—not as hard to use but not as blink-proof. Figures 5 and 6 are made by Volk, but they are similar to the various Mainster lenses manufactured by Ocular Instruments. (Courtesy of Volk Optical.)

Unfortunately, these lenses can be frustrating. One begins with the preconceived notion that one simply needs to slap on the lens and one will immediately see broad vistas of retina. Just like the first time you tried to ski, snowboard or ice skate, however, the reality is a bit different from the expectations. Strive to overcome your initial disappointment and keep trying—the necessary moves will become automatic with practice, and you will soon become a contact lens Jedi.

Indirect lenses require a much more dynamic approach than the direct view lenses. At all times you need to try to keep a straight line from the patient's retina through the lens and slit lamp and onto your fovea—something that is much easier said than done with this class of lens. (In reality the optics are more complicated, but the straight-line approach is a good mental goal to start with.)

Even if you can get the patient lined up to obtain the best view, you need to continually coordinate movements between the slit lamp, the lens and the eye in subtle ways. This can be very frustrating at first because it feels like you will never succeed. It helps to break this process down into a few separate moves until it becomes automatic...

You have to take full advantage of all the different ways you can shift the lens around the eye. A common problem is not being able to get a good view of what you want to see with both of your eyes—a classic sign that you are not as lined up as you think you are. Try moving the lens in a circle or a cone—this is a handy way of scanning for the best line of sight (Figure 7). Remember, you have to be ready to follow any move you make with the lens by shifting the position of the slit lamp. This last point is really important. An understandable novice move is to concentrate on moving just the lens, because it is difficult enough to manipulate the lens without letting it slide off the eye. However, if you move only the lens without following that inverted image with the slit lamp, you will never get a good view. It helps to affix your lens hand to the patient by spreading your fourth and fifth fingers onto the side of the patient's face or by putting the back of those fingers on the patient's cheek—this gives you more stability and you don't have to exert as much brain power worrying about keeping the lens on the eye. This way you can better concentrate exclusively on moving the lens and the slit lamp as needed in order to get the best view.

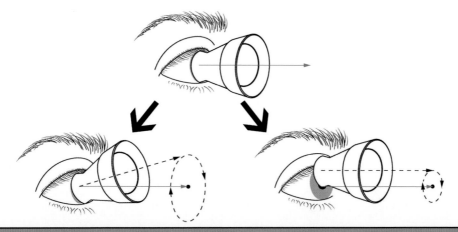

Figure 7. This figure shows slightly different ways of moving the lens around the eye in order to find the best view. These are an exaggeration of the movements required—the real moves are much more subtle. The top image shows a perfectly lined up lens, but this almost never happens spontaneously. The quickest way to find the best view is to rotate the lens around the presumed visual axis. The lower left image shows that you can rotate the axis of the lens so that it creates a cone. In this case, the part of the lens on the eye moves just a little, and the part of the lens facing the slit lamp circles around a lot. The lower right image shows that you can move the lens such that its axis creates a cylinder, with the entire lens moving in the same circular pattern. In reality, you will rapidly learn to combine both moves to scan for the best view—but it helps to realize that each one of these motions will give a slightly different effect, which may come in handy in different circumstances. Remember to follow any moves you make with the lens with corresponding movement of the slit lamp; otherwise, you are wasting your time. Note that if you still can't get a great view, you need to recheck where the patient is looking—they may be rotating their eye out of reach.

Don't worry if you aren't getting a perfect view at first—the goal here is to just see what you want to see with both eyes at the same time. Once you can do this reliably, it is time for some real finesse: the "Five Point Palm Exploding Heart Technique" of lens wrassling, if you will. It is similar to the technique mentioned in the section on direct lenses, wherein you use the lens to torque the eye in different directions. Sometimes, you will do this by translating the entire lens in one direction, and sometimes you will do this in a more subtle way: by slightly rotating the lens around its midpoint (kind of like adjusting the pitch of an airplane). Both moves will slightly change the visual axis of the lens and will slightly rotate the eye at the same time, with the goal being a much more favorable view. (If this is an obtuse paragraph, look at Figure 8, where the proverbial thousand words await). By the way, if you are having a lot of trouble getting a view, even with all these moves, go back and double check where the patient's fixation is. There is no way, at least at first, that you can get a good view if the patient is rolling their eye up in their head—you will never line things up. (There will be more discussion about enlisting the patient's cooperation in Chapter 7.)

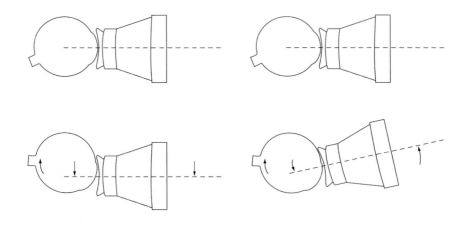

Figure 8. These are exaggerated images of moves you can make to fine-tune your view with an indirect contact lens. On the left, you are moving the entire lens in one direction and keeping the axis of the lens parallel as you move it. At the same time, you are "pulling" the eye with you to try to line up the axis of the lens with whatever you need to see. The image on the right shows a slightly different way of doing the same thing; here, you are torquing the lens through its center as you also rotate the eye, so the axis of the lens is tilting. Both moves accomplish the same goal, but they will give you slightly different views depending on the orientation of the patient's eye. You will rapidly learn to use a combination of both moves to get the best view, but it helps to consciously try them out at first—with practice, your brain will create a macro that automatically moves the lens into the best position using whatever move is necessary.

How do you know which way to tilt the lens to get the best view? At first, you may need to use very gross and even random movements to get a rough view of what you want to see. As things get fine-tuned, you can sometimes let Dr. Sturm and his conoid guide you. Look at your aiming beam. Unless you are a natural, it is likely the aiming beam will be some sort of smeared oval, suggesting that you are out of alignment to a tiny degree. The long axis of the oval tells you which way to rock the lens. Say the long axis is vertical—then tilt the lens up and down around its center and watch the beam—it will shift around and tighten up into a circle as you become more perfectly aligned. Sometimes you have to be more aggressive and move the whole lens up or down to follow the long axis of the aiming beam and then fine-tune with a little gentle tilting. Sometimes you can rotate the eye with the lens as you tilt it and get to your goal even faster. Don't forget to follow your lens moves with the slit lamp, although as you get closer and closer to a good view, you usually do not need to move the microscope as much.

Sadly, there will still be a lot of hit and miss, and you will find that you have to keep iterating and reiterating all of these moves to get in focus and stay in focus. First, get lined up grossly by circling the visual axis. Then try some tilting to offset the long axis of the aiming beam—then do a little more circling and tilting, and ultimately you will be rewarded with a lovely panoramic view that makes treatment very easy. Eventually, all these actions will be internalized and, as with indirect ophthalmoscopy, you will begin to automatically make the right moves without thinking. Just don't give up and do keep trying.

You will need different indirect lenses depending on whether you want to treat the macula or the periphery. Macular lenses don't get out very far, but they give you a nice stereoscopic view of the posterior pole. Wide-field lenses, on the other hand, will let you see much more of the periphery (you will have to ignore the impressive marketing names such as Ultra-Quadro-Magnoview, etc., and ask about the field of view as measured in degrees in order to find out exactly how much of the periphery you are supposed to see). The wide-field lenses will allow you to see the posterior pole, but the view is nowhere near as stereoscopic as that obtained with a lens designed to view the macula. Furthermore, there tend to be a lot of light reflexes when viewing the central retina with a wide-field lens—which make viewing the macula problematic. (Sometimes you can minimize the reflexes by moving your slit beam a bit off axis and/or by decreasing the size of the slit lamp beam.)

Finally, the wider the field of view, the more the lens will magnify the size of your spot, which means that it is hard to safely place small focal burns in the macula with such a lens. (See the next blue box.) All this is why there is not one indirect lens that can be used to treat both the periphery and the macula. Predictably, manufacturers have created a host of different indirect lenses that cover the whole spectrum from very wide-field to very focal macular viewing. As mentioned in the beginning of the chapter, you may want to get comfortable with just one macular and one wide-field lens, and then you can decide whether you want all the more nuanced lenses that are available.

Indirect lenses and spot size

With the direct view lenses, the spot you set on your laser is pretty much the size you will get on the retina, give or take a few microns. The indirect lenses, however, will change the spot size in a manner proportional to the field of view. For instance, a really wide-field lens, like the Mainster 165, can almost double the diameter of your spot setting (a 100-micron spot on the laser turns into a 200-micron spot on the retina). Indirect lenses designed for the macula tend to deliver spot sizes that are closer to the actual laser setting, but they will still vary depending on the width of the field. Some "high-power" macular lenses can actually make the delivered spot smaller relative to the laser setting.

This becomes very important if you are trying to deliver a specific dose of laser energy to a given area (such as with photodynamic therapy for macular degeneration). It is less important in the setting of diabetic lasers, because you will be titrating the energy dose yourself, based on the uptake you see as you do the laser.

Nevertheless, you need to be aware of the effect your chosen lens has on the delivered spot size—lens manufacturers always include this information with each lens and publish it on their websites. If you are trying to, say, follow the Diabetic Retinopathy Study guidelines in terms of spot size and number, you need to realize that if you are using a wide-field lens and you set your laser to 500 microns, you will be placing much bigger burns than you want. Alternatively, if you switch from a wide-field lens to a macular lens, you will make your spot size much smaller. If you do not adjust your power accordingly, you can burn a hole in the retina.

There are two situations in which the wider-field indirect lenses can be useful beyond their ability to allow easy panretinal photocoagulation (PRP). First, if the patient has media opacities, such as a central posterior subcapsular cataract, you may be able to use these lenses to treat the posterior pole. They tend to "reach around" the opacity better than indirect lenses designed for the macula, and certainly better than direct lenses. As mentioned above, you need to do this carefully because you will be creating a large diffused spot, but it may be better than nothing in difficult situations.

The other situation in which the wide-field indirect lenses are extremely useful is when you are looking for retinal breaks in pseudophakic patients. The prismatic effect of the edge of the intraocular lens will often keep you from seeing the far periphery with a direct view lens. A wide-field lens allows better visualization, and such a lens can allow you to find and treat a peripheral tear without the need for a binocular indirect laser or cryotherapy. This last point is a bit off-topic for a book on diabetic retinopathy, but it is good to know.

One other weird thing about wide-field indirect contact lenses: The nature of their optics is such that the irradiance can be higher through the patient's lens and cornea than at the retina. This effect is usually insignificant, but it can become a problem with huge (greater than 500-micron) spot sizes—although one would usually not use such large spots. The problem is that if there are a lot of lens opacities the high irradiance through the anterior segment can cause lenticular burns. Corneal burns can also occur with even smaller spots if there is pigment on the surface of the cornea or if you trap an eyelash or mascara under the contact lens. Furthermore, it is likely you won't realize that these burns are occurring because you are not able to easily visualize the anterior segment through an indirect-view contact lens. This is why you need to stop and take the contact lens off and look at the front of the eye if you find that your view of the retina is clouding up. These problems are relatively unusual with modern treatment techniques, but it is good to remember that Murphy's Law can extend far beyond the retina that you are working on. (There will be more on this in Chapter 16, discussing complications.)

What specific lenses should be in your toolbox for retinal lasers? It's a matter of personal taste. There are two main companies that make lenses: Volk and Ocular Instruments. They both make great laser lenses and their product lines tend to be roughly equivalent (although the manufacturers themselves might disagree). They both have return policies, so you can try out different lenses and decide what works for you. Here are some suggestions for a basic lineup:

1. A Goldmann three mirror can do everything reasonably well, but it may take longer to do a treatment and it is not as versatile as separate lenses. Nevertheless, if you can get only one lens, this is the one to have. If you have been good and the Retina Bunny is going to bring you more than one lens, then please read on...

2. A general-purpose indirect macular lens such as the Volk Area Centralis or the Ocular Instruments Standard Mainster will likely become your main lens for focal and grid laser. There are plenty of variations, so you can pretty much choose exactly how much field of view you want—but don't get a field of view that is too big, because the wider the field of view, the harder it is to treat the macula accurately.

3. A pancake lens for an extra-crisp view of the macula (i.e., for diagnosis or very accurate focal treatment of microaneurysms in cooperative patients). Examples would be the Yanuzzi lens by Ocular Instruments or the Fundus 20 by Volk.

4. A wide-field indirect lens for PRPs such as the Mainster 165 by Ocular Instruments or the Super Quad 160 by Volk.

References and Suggested Reading

Mainster MA, Crossman JL, Erickson PJ, Heacock GL. Retinal laser lenses: magnification, spot size, and field of view. Br J Ophthalmol 1990;74:177-9.

Folk JC, Pulido JS. Laser photocoagulation of the retina and choroid. San Francisco: American Academy of Ophthalmology, 1997.

L'Esperance FA. Ophthalmic lasers, 3rd ed. St. Louis: Mosby, 1989.

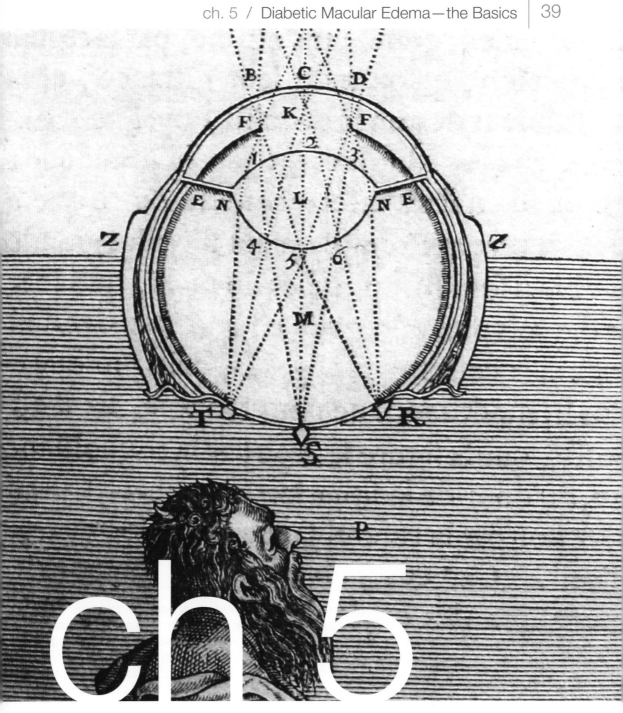

ch5

Diabetic Macular Edema—the Basics

DOING THE EXAM in 2-D

This chapter discusses macular edema resulting from microvascular leakage around the posterior pole. Basically, diabetes turns the retinal capillaries into the vascular equivalent of leaky old garden hoses. The result is that patients develop microaneurysms, hard exudates, and hemorrhages in varying amounts. If there is a lot of leakage from the damaged vessels, then the retina will swell up like a sponge. If this swelling builds up in and around the center of vision, then permanent damage can occur, and the goal is to identify swelling and treat it well before this happens.

Besides causing leaky blood vessels, diabetes can also just kill off blood vessels. Most of the time, there is a combination of both problems—vascular leakage and capillary death. In some patients, the destruction of blood vessels is the predominant problem, and this is referred to as capillary dropout or macular ischemia. This is always bad and it can cause marked vision loss; so far there is no treatment other than prevention with good systemic control and by trying to address any treatable leakage. Although capillary dropout can cause retinal edema at first as a result of ischemia, the end result is a thinned-out retina. It usually requires a fluorescein angiogram to identify this problem, although it can be inferred if patients have marked vision loss and an atrophic-appearing fovea. (Figure 7 is an example of capillary dropout around the fovea.)

Unless the patient is truly unlucky, ischemia is usually not a predominant feature in the early stages of diabetic macular edema. Instead, vascular leakage tends to be the initial finding. Because this leakage is very treatable, it is crucial to be able to identify the clinical signs that indicate the beginnings of damage. At the very start of your career it is exciting to simply be able to see these findings—your first direct glimpse of a disease hard at work. However, once you master the mechanics of examining the fundus it is easy to become jaded about spotting the signs of retinopathy. Try not to let this happen. You can get a lot of clues about a patient's situation just by looking carefully at each of the various manifestations.

For instance, you are no doubt aware that most intraretinal hemorrhages in diabetic retinopathy are blot-shaped because they stem from broken capillaries in the outer retinal layers, where the neurons are all jumbled together. As a result, the hemorrhage seeps out radially like a drop of food coloring on a paper towel. Flame-shaped hemorrhages occur when capillaries break in the more superficial nerve fiber layer, where the linear arrangement of the axons spreads the blood lengthwise rather than in all directions.

You may think that you are too cool to care about this second-year medical student stuff. You aren't. If a patient has an excessive number of flame-shaped hemorrhages and/or dot-blot hemorrhages, you should worry about the presence of additional vascular risk factors that are not well controlled. The most likely culprit would be superimposed hypertension, but you might also see this with progressive renal failure or anemia. Many such patients also have poor compliance—usually due to a combination of lack of motivation, lack of insurance or lack of a motivated primary-care doctor. Based on a few red smears it is possible to make massive inferences about everything from a patient's creatinine to their socioeconomic status—and your deductions and consequent actions can have a dramatic impact on how the patient responds to your ministrations.

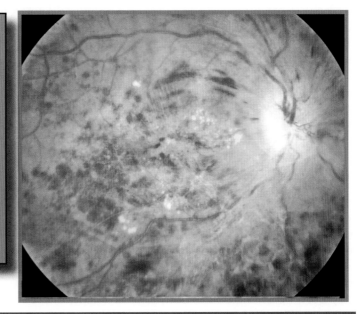

Figure 1. A patient with macular edema and multiple hemorrhages. This patient had severe hypertension, early renal failure with secondary anemia and had been uninsured and unable to afford an eye exam until he could no longer function. You can infer a lot from a retina.

In Chapter 1, it was pointed out that we all went into ophthalmology because taking care of an entire patient is not our bag, man. If we could get the eye mailed to us—without the attached patient—that would be fine. However, if you see worrisome hemorrhages, it is definitely time to dust off those atrophied clinical skills and check a blood pressure. Right there in the lane. While you are at it, you should also order a CBC, hemoglobin A1c and renal studies if no one has done them lately. These tests will identify significant problems much faster than a referral letter will, and the results will jumpstart the patient's care. Oh yeah, you might also help save their life (which is a nice break from a day full of "better one, better two"). The point is to try to take advantage of all the information the fundus is willing to give you. If you look, but do not see, you will be failing to treat the patient's eye properly (and also be very un-Zen).

Another hemorrhagic nuance occurs in patients who are taking Coumadin. These patients will often have many more hemorrhages in the retina relative to their overall degree of retinopathy (in other words, they have more hemorrhages than you would expect, given the number of microaneurysms and non-hemorrhagic vascular changes that you see). All these hemorrhages may have varying sizes and unusual shapes. Make sure that your patients that are on this rat poison are really getting their levels checked; you will find occasional patients that are not being monitored properly. A more complete discussion of this drug in terms of diabetic retinopathy is found in Chapter 25.

Cotton wool spots are another fundus finding that can tell you a lot about the patient. These used to be considered very important in terms of predicting future proliferative disease, but this has been disproven (which makes one wonder what other "facts" will be disproved in the future, which, in turn, makes one glad this book is produced with software and not woodcuts). A few scattered cotton wool spots are to be expected, and individual spots may last for several months. However, if there are a lot of cotton wool spots or if crops of new lesions appear rather quickly, it may signal problems with hypertension, renal failure, or hematologic abnormalities. Never forget that patients are also allowed to get completely unrelated problems, and it is always possible that a patient with lots of cotton wool spots may have an additional disease such as AIDS, retinal vasculitis or radiation retinopathy. Given the overall sturm and drang of diabetic retinopathy, it may be difficult to dissect out the presence of these other diseases unless you remember to think of them in the first place. (Check Chapter 26 for the full scoop on this.)

When actively studying hemorrhages and cotton wool spots, the Renaissance Retina Observer also inspects the hard exudate situation. Hard exudates begin to appear as more and more leakage occurs. You can think of them as high-water marks—the serum bathtub rings that outline where the retina is desperately trying to suck the abnormal fluid back into the capillaries and the leftover protein and lipid congeal into little yellow lumps. These lumps may be all over, but often they show up on the border between the healthy and damaged retina. Large amounts of hard exudates should always suggest the possibility of hyperlipidemia, so be sure to inform their medical doctor. Patients should be trained to consider their lipid profile to be as important as their blood pressure and hemoglobin A1c. Tight lipid control is a little-recognized aspect of total diabetic care, at least in the ophthalmic community, and pointing out to the patient that you can see "all those little fatty deposits" in their retina may be more of a motivator for healthy living than weeks of diabetic education classes.

There is always something a bit mysterious, even to sophisticated patients, about having someone look into one's eye and being told that damage is visible. Sometimes, this can be a very effective tool for encouraging patients to take better care of themselves. Sometimes, however, it can be very depressing for patients to hear this—and you need to be sensitive to this as well. This is a good reason why it really is better that we don't get the eyes mailed to us. Chapter 20 will elaborate on issues like this a bit more.

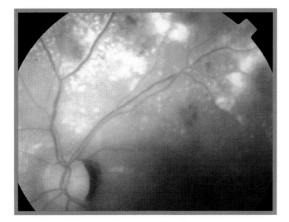

Figure 2. This kind of extensive hard exudate formation, especially along peripheral vessels, is very suggestive of hyperlipidemia.

DOING THE EXAM in 3-D

Having developed some familiarity with the two-dimensional findings of background diabetic retinopathy, it is now time to go 3-D by looking for macular edema. Macular edema may be "focal," which means that small, localized areas of microaneurysms create circumscribed areas of thickening, often surrounded by rings of hard exudates. Macular edema may also be diffuse, involving larger areas of the posterior pole and arising not only from microaneurysms, but also from diffuse capillary leakage throughout the vascular bed. Usually, there is a combination of both types of leakage.

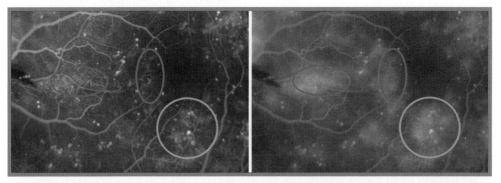

Figure 3. An example of different types of leakage. The green circles show areas where focal leakage from several microaneurysms predominates. The red ovals show areas where diffuse leakage from capillary beds predominates. Most areas are a mix of both.

Occasionally, diffuse macular edema may be difficult to diagnose because the whole retina is uniformly thickened, and unless you have a sense of "normal" thickening on clinical examination, the diagnosis may not be obvious. Most of the time the associated vision loss will point you in the right direction. Of course, your ocular coherence tomography machine (OCT) is perfect in this situation, but not everyone will have access to such high-tech stuff, so do try to perfect your clinical exam. (There is more on OCT at the end of the chapter.)

Perfecting Your Clinical Exam

It is absolutely crucial that you take the time to put a diagnostic contact lens on these patients, especially in the early stages of your diabetic retinopathy treatment career. There is simply not enough axial magnification with the indirect slit lamp lenses (such as a 90- or 78-diopter lens) to really allow you to get a sense of how succulent the retina can become.* It helps to visualize individual microaneurysms, hemorrhages and exudates and to note their height above the pigment epithelium at various places in the posterior pole. You can get a very definite feel for how thick the retina is by going back and forth between flatter, more peripheral areas and more swollen central areas. A thin off-axis slit beam helps somewhat in bringing out the three-dimensional structure, but nothing helps as much as just getting the contact lens on the patient and doing the exam multiple times.

It is also very instructive to look at a recent fluorescein angiogram as you are examining the patient (and definitely when you are performing laser treatment). Carefully study each little lesion in the fundus and compare it to the angiographic appearance. You will note that many of the tiny red dots that you assume to be microaneurysms on clinical examination actually do not light up at all on the angiogram. These are simply dot hemorrhages and you may be wasting laser spots (and the patient's non-expendable RPE) if you shoot at them. Worse, these dot hemorrhages may readily take up laser energy and change color very easily—one of the criteria for successful treatment—and you may feel like you have done a great job, but you may simply have toasted valuable portions of the patient's nerve fiber layer. On the other hand, there will be many real microaneurysms that are invisible on your initial clinical exam but will then become apparent when you trace their location on the angiogram and track them down in the patient's fundus. These represent your true targets. Chapter 8 will cover all of this at length, but you have to know what you are looking for by doing the drills discussed here.

After tracing all of these lesions out on the angiogram and then finding them in the fundus on several patients, you will find that you are better and better at identifying these tiny lesions without an angiogram. Even if you try this only two or three times, you will be amazed at how your clinical skills will improve (and

---

*Remember, a 60-diopter lens does have more axial magnification, but it is hard for even an experienced user to stuff both visual axes through this lens and the patient's pupil and have both images be in-focus enough to get a good view. Best to work with a contact lens to build up experience, and then you may want to try a lens of this power—although as you improve your exam you probably won't need the extra axial magnification, anyway.

how your lasers will be more effective and less damaging). The result is better patient care and more efficient use of your valuable time—everybody wins!

The point is that you really need to get a feel for how "unobvious" diabetic retinopathy can be in order to fine-tune your ability to treat it properly, and the only way to develop your skills is to take the time to compare the fluorescein to the patient on a microscopic level before you take on the responsibility of treating the disease with laser.

Stereo Photographs

In the days when retinal photographers used film, it was common to obtain stereo photos of fundus pathology. You should ask around, because even in the most digital photography departments, they may have some old stereo slides of diabetic retinopathy in the files. Another good source of stereo photos can be found in some of the older, beat-up textbooks in the back of your departmental library—especially the ones that have the little discs and 3-D viewer in the back. For instance, Gass's *Stereoscopic Atlas of Macular Diseases* is so fantastic it can induce LSD flashbacks.

Stereo photos and fluoresceins are a beautiful way to get a sense of what is meant by the term "retinal thickening"—if you are having a hard time figuring out just what you are supposed to see, it will just take a few seconds of browsing stereo pics and you will understand. Note that stereo imaging with the fundus camera is more exaggerated than on clinical examination, and do not expect your patients to have the kind dramatic elevation that is seen on good stereo photographs. It will, however, give you a very good idea of what to train your eye to look for.

BUT ENOUGH ON THE EXAM on to the disease

All of the above is about being able to identify macular edema in general, but the real enemy is known as "clinically significant diabetic macular edema" (CSDME). This term is reserved for findings that indicate a very high risk of progressive visual loss. The exact criteria for CSDME should be burned into your brain at this point in your career, but here it is for reference:

Criteria for Clinically Significant Diabetic Macular Edema

> 1. Retinal thickening within 500 microns of the center of the fovea.

> 2. Hard exudates within 500 microns of the center of the fovea that are associated with some degree of surrounding retinal thickening. (You should take a moment to ponder this second criterion. Both hard exudates and microaneurysms may be present without retinal thickening and, if there isn't any thickening, there definitely isn't any CSDME.)

3. One disc area of thickening, part of which is within one disc diameter of the center (or, to paraphrase Edgar Allen Poe, a disc within a disc).

The whole reason for defining CSDME this way is because the Early Treatment of Diabetic Retinopathy Study (ETDRS)[1] showed that unless a patient actually has CSDME, the rate of vision loss was so low that there was hardly any treatment effect. (It is a tribute to the genius of the pioneers of diabetic treatment that they could define the disease in absolutely the most useful way—and do it before they even started the study!)

On the other hand, if patients do have CSDME, then treatment results in about a 50% decrease in the incidence of moderate visual loss at the three-year mark (Figure 4). Moderate vision loss was defined as doubling at the visual angle (i.e., 20/30 going to 20/60). Preventing this much vision loss is truly a Good Thing, and should rev you up for reading the chapters that follow.

> I stand amid the roar
> Of a surf-tormented shore,
> And I hold within my hand
> Grains of the golden sand—
> How few! yet how they creep
> Through my fingers to the deep,
> While I weep—while I weep!
> O God! can I not grasp
> Them with a tighter clasp?
> O God! can I not save
> One from the pitiless wave?
> Is all that we see or seem
> But a dream within a dream?
>
> (This is just the second stanza. That guy could write...)

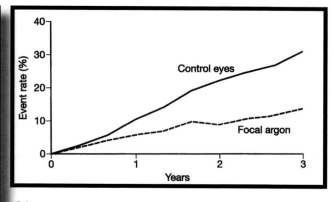

Figure 4. The classic graph from the ETDRS showing the effect of treatment on the rate of moderate vision loss from macular edema. (Photocoagulation for diabetic macular edema. Early Treatment Diabetic Retinopathy Study report number 1. Arch Ophthalmol 1985;103:1796-806. Copyright © American Medical Association, 1985. All rights reserved.)

Of course, like everything else in life, the decision to treat a patient is usually more complex than deciding that someone has "crossed the line" into CSDME and firing away. Here are some factors to consider:

1. What is the patient's systemic status? A well controlled patient, with disease that is far away from the fovea (i.e., at the outer limits of the disc within a disc rule), may do very well with just observation. Such patients may actually heal themselves and end up not needing treatment. Follow them closely, though, to be sure they don't progress.

2. Conversely, treat a poorly controlled patient more aggressively to try to keep them out of trouble. Be aware that these patients tend to go downhill even if the treatment works well, and this creates nuances that need to be addressed with the informed consent. The next chapter elaborates on this.

3. Be careful with disease close to the fovea. There is a balance to be struck in these situations—if you have to risk torching a patient's perifoveal vision with a laser, it may be better to do nothing. Mild disease in this location can be very indolent, and the patient may actually be better off in the long run without intervention. An additional factor to consider in this situation is whether there is a role for intravitreal therapy in order to avoid treatment at the edge of the fovea. Chapter 11 tries to discuss this, but because there are no clear-cut guidelines at present, you will need to get a sense of how your local retinal community wants you to deal with such patients.

4. Is there a reversible factor that is contributing to the edema? For instance, some patients with renal failure and fluid retention will lose their edema once they are on dialysis. Or, edema present in pregnant patients may resolve without treatment after they deliver.

A lot of the above issues, as well as others, will be discussed in the chapters that cover what to do when you actually decide to treat someone. For now, just concentrate on doing the best exam you can and becoming familiar with how to call CSDME. Oh, and one other thing…

DIPLOMACY FOR DUMMIES
Something to Not Do as You Begin to Study Diabetic Fundi

If you are examining a diabetic that has already had macular laser—especially old-school treatment that tended to be heavy—you may be surprised about the amount of laser spots that are visible. You have to be very careful about how you refer to these previous laser spots.

For instance, early in your career you may be excited that you have managed to identify spots in the first place and you may gleefully carry on about all the scars that you can see with your whiz-bang 90-diopter skills. Or you may develop the tendency we all have: to try to make oneself look good by pointing out how others have done poorly by commenting about "all those spots back there"—vaguely implying that you are way too chill to drop that many hits into someone's macula.

Avoid doing these things.

First of all, if you are seeing a patient years after a treatment, it is very hard to comment wisely because you did not see what the fundus looked like at the time and you don't have any idea how bad the patient might have been without the laser. Also, remember that if you refer uncharitably to previous laser treatment, it may just be a matter of time before what goes around comes around and your laser spots are being disrespected.

More importantly, patients can be very frightened to learn about "laser scars" in the back of their eye because at some level they may imagine crazed doctors trying to carve up their vision in order to pay for Hummers. They also will assume that any vision problems they have are due to the scars; they usually do not entirely understand that the lasers have, in fact, managed to save what vision they have.

The problem is that when patients draw incorrect conclusions about the effect of laser treatment on their vision, they can become very reluctant to undergo laser treatment by anyone, including your own bad self, when they desperately need it. As subsequent chapters will discuss, it can be hard enough to get a patient to return for follow up, and you don't want to contribute to the problem by carrying on about oodles and scads of spots.

This warning also applies to any primary-eye-care practitioners who may be reading this. It is not uncommon for patients to return from their optometrist somewhat upset because, with the best of intentions, the OD has referred to 'all those scars back there'. Even a casual remark like that can potentially interfere with appropriate follow up. If you are going to talk about laser scars, be sure to remind the patient why they are there in the first place—and where their vision would have ended up without intervention. Perhaps it is better to use the term "treatment" rather than "laser scars" in order to describe the findings.

In fact, carefully placed laser spots usually have nothing to do with a patient's symptoms. For instance, many diabetic patients will complain of microscotomas around the center of their vision as they age—often manifesting as missing parts of words or letters. It is very easy for them (and you) to assume that these scotomas are from laser scars. However, most of the time laser spots are well outside the area where they could interfere with reading. Instead, the "spots" they are seeing are actually caused by capillary dropout around the fovea (Figure 5). If you casually blame the symptoms on the laser, you will have unjustly maligned one of your colleagues and you will be risking the patient's compliance forever. You are managing to do two really bad things at once without even trying.

Of course, there is no question that previous scars can enlarge over time, and you will see patients that were treated years ago with very heavy treatment and who have undergone scar expansion that can look rather frightening.[2] Although many times these patients are surprisingly asymptomatic for such scars, some patients will clearly have vision loss due to this process. If you feel that this is indeed the case, then you have to call it as you see it, but it still helps to remind the patient that without treatment, their vision would likely be far worse.

As an aside, here is something else to be aware of. When hard exudates build up in the fovea, they can sometimes leave a focal depigmented scar when they fade away. This scar can look for all the world like someone placed a laser spot right in the fovea. A classic tyro move is to tell the patient that their fovea was lasered when this was not the case at all. This results in a whole bunch of needless grief and once again manages to unjustly malign a colleague and alienate a patient in one fell swoop. Just be careful what you say.

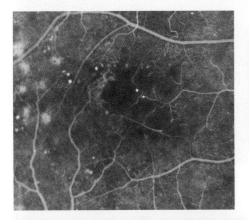

Figure 5. A patient complaining of difficulty seeing parts of words when reading. The laser scars are far away from areas involved in reading. The paracentral scotomas are from the capillary dropout and are not iatrogenic.

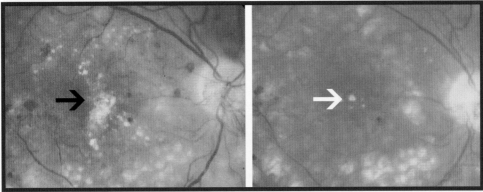

Figure 6. Hard exudates can build up in the fovea, as in the picture on the left (black arrow). When the exudates resolve, they can leave an area of focal depigmentation that can look just like a laser scar, as in the photo on the right (white arrow). No one lasered this fovea, so don't even think about freaking the patient out by calling this a laser spot. By the way, note the expansion of the real laser scars everywhere else.

OPTICAL COHERENCE TOMOGRAPHY OCT

OCT has revolutionized our ability to visualize the architecture of the retina, and it can be extremely valuable for evaluating and following patients with diabetic retinopathy. As with fluorescein angiography, this review will assume that the reader has some familiarity with OCT testing already and will not cover finer points of how the test works or interpretation. Fortunately, the data provided by OCT testing is fairly intuitive and fits right in with one's basic understanding of retinal anatomy. This section will refer primarily to scans produced by the Zeiss Stratus, which is perhaps the most common OCT machine.

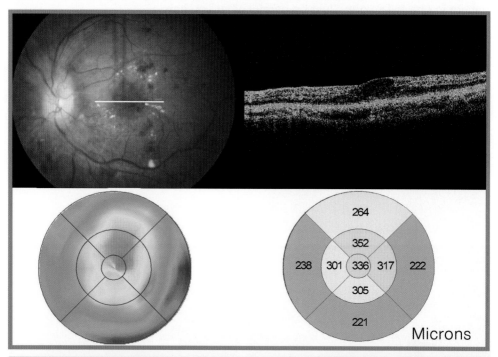

Figure 7. Standard OCT findings. The line on the color photo indicates the cut of the B scan (upper left). The B scan shows retinal thickening centrally (upper right). The lower left is the topographic retinal thickness map generated by averaging between the different B scans; it shows a focus of retinal swelling in and above the fovea. The lower right gives the average numeric thickness of nine sections of the scan. Really, if this is all new to you, please grab an OCT book. (Zeiss makes a basic one that you may be able to get for free—see the references at the end of the chapter.)

There are a few things to be aware of, however. OCT testing comes in two flavors: the individual B scans that give you cross-sectional anatomy of the retina, and the various macular thickness protocols that give you the equivalent of a topographic map of an entire region of the retina. However, if you are simply looking at the topographic map, you can be fooled because the topographic map is generated by "smearing" together six individual B scans in order to extrapolate the retinal surface. The computer then tries to recognize the RPE and the retinal nerve fiber layer in order to calculate the overall retinal volume. It is possible for the computer to misinterpret the different retinal layers and give you information that is misleading—this is known as a boundary line error. Boundary line errors are especially common if the signal is weak due to a poorly done study or media opacity. Figure 4 shows the characteristic appearance of the effect of boundary errors on the topographic map.

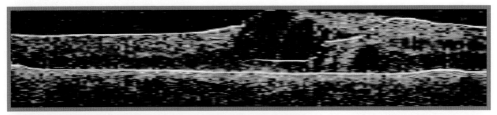

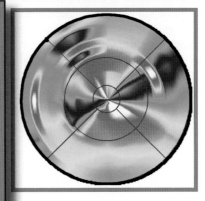

Figure 8. OCT boundary error. Note that the white lines do not follow the actual retinal architecture (above). This usually happens with very abnormal morphology and low signal strength (in this case the signal was attenuated by a vitreous hemorrhage). If you don't look at what the computer is doing, you can be very much misled, although you can usually get an idea that something is wrong when you look at the retinal thickness map (right). When it looks like something you made at the spin-art booth at your elementary school fair, with weird hourglass colors and everything, you can bet that the computer misread the image.

Ideally, you should study at least three of the separate B scans to get a sense of whether the boundary lines are screwed up and to get an idea of the morphology in different areas. If you are only looking at just one horizontal B scan, you are missing a lot of useful data. For instance, Figure 9 shows a situation where one cut has a little bit of retinal thickening and an epiretinal membrane, but does not appear particularly ominous. A cut 90 degrees away shows a traction retinal detachment encroaching on the fovea.

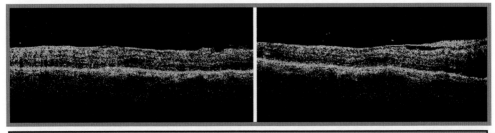

Figure 9. This is why you need to look at more than one cut of the OCT. The left shows some retinal thickening and an epiretinal membrane—no big deal. The right is 90 degrees away, showing a much more ominous tractional detachment extending toward the fovea. Yes, you should have seen this on your clinical exam, but sometimes the clinical exam is subtle and the point is that you never want to be reassured by only one cut from the OCT—in the same way that you would never treat a routine glaucoma patient based on one pressure measurement.

You should also take a look at some of the options available when it comes to using the OCT machine. You should understand what the technicians are doing and be aware of the different fixation parameters, line cuts, image processing techniques and levels of resolution available. You can even—gasp—do the scan yourself if you have a patient who has an area of concern and you are not seeing what you need to see on the OCT cuts provided.

Although traditional OCT machines acquire data by performing one slice at a time (time domain OCT), newer machines can examine an entire region of the retina with one scan (spectral domain or Fourier domain OCT). Subtle areas of pathology can be missed if they fall in between the scans on a time domain machine, and newer machines are much better able to identify abnormal anatomy, such as early vitreous traction. However, the technology is expensive and tends to Hoover up vast amounts of computer memory, so such machines are usually found in specialist's offices. They can be helpful in difficult cases, so if you have a time domain machine like the Stratus remember that some patients may benefit from the next generation of machines. He who dies with the most toys...

OCT & DME That You Don't See

There is no question that one can sooner identify retinal thickening with OCT testing than with clinical examination. What is not clear is whether this has therapeutic implications. You have to remember that all of the studies looking at the treatment of diabetic macular edema were based on how the retina appears clinically. If the OCT shows thickening that one cannot see on clinical exam, it is not known for sure whether such patients benefit from treatment.

If you do not see any obvious thickening, then it has been suggested that about two-thirds of the time the edema will not progress to clinically significant disease.[3] This can become hard to call, though, because once the OCT brings something to your attention, you can start to hallucinate some thickening. You have to be intellectually honest and promise not to manufacture clinically significant disease in your head just because you want to treat a retina.

Ultimately, deciding whether to treat such patients is an art-of-medicine thing—there are a lot of variables that may play into the decision. If the process appears to be progressive, then it may be reasonable to get in some early treatment to head off trouble. This is especially true if the thickening appears to be due to a few small microaneurysms that are away from the fovea and can be safely treated. On the other hand, if the patient does not have any symptoms and is systemically well-controlled, very early edema will often resolve without the need for treatment (i.e., without the need for putting permanent spots in and around the patient's fovea).

It is also important to remember that, in general, the treatment of diabetic macular edema that is not fovea-threatening is never an emergency. It is reasonable to simply re-examine the patient in six to eight weeks and monitor the changes (this interval may vary depending on their disease and your level of concern). If nothing else, being able to use the pretty OCT colors to show asymptomatic patients how they are developing evidence of their diabetes can sometimes serve to motivate patients better than a ton of handouts.

Another extremely important use of OCT is the ability to identify problems with the vitreoretinal interface that can contribute to persistent edema. Although a careful clinical exam can usually suggest the presence of a subtle epiretinal membrane or taut cortical vitreous, abnormalities like this tend to become immediately obvious with OCT testing. This is useful when you have a patient with persistent edema and decreasing vision in spite of laser. If you identify subtle traction, then you know that such a patient should be referred to your friendly neighborhood retina specialist, rather than given 300 more laser spots in a fruitless attempt to seal leaks in a retina that is slowly being pulled apart by the vitreous. There will be much more on this in subsequent chapters.

But I Don't Have an OCT…

Are you going to go to Retina Hell if you try to manage diabetics without an OCT? There are plenty of places around the world where it is simply not possible to generate the capital to obtain an OCT machine. Fortunately, the majority of studies about treating diabetic retinopathy are totally based on clinical examination. Moreover, a careful observer can usually identify—or at least suspect—the kinds of problems that an OCT machine can find. The only difference is that the OCT makes detecting such findings effortless.

On the other hand, most retinal specialists would say that having an OCT is the standard of care when it comes to managing complex diabetic patients. As a result, if you think you can get an OCT it is a good idea to obtain one. The machine will likely keep you from doing the wrong thing to diabetics, and there are lots of other good things it can do. (Perhaps the most useful is the ability to identify subtle macular problems prior to cataract surgery, such as a diaphanous epiretinal membrane. You do not want a patient that is paying you the big bucks for a multifocal implant to be surprised by post-op pucker.)

If you can't get an OCT, do not worry. Just keep on improving your exam and watching for the kinds of things discussed in this book that can mess you up—almost always, a high index of suspicion and a careful contact lens exam will keep you out of the land of permanent-vision-loss-because-you-missed-something. That particular location is not a happy place to be.

Of course, things start to get complicated if you *might* be able to obtain an OCT machine but you really need something more important, like a faster car. Only you and the Great Ophthalmic Court in the Sky can decide the answer to that one…

References and Suggested Reading

1.   Photocoagulation for diabetic macular edema. Early Treatment Diabetic Retinopathy Study report number 1. Early Treatment Diabetic Retinopathy Study research group. Arch Ophthalmol 1985;103:1796-806.

2.   Maeshima K, Utsugi-Sutoh N, Otani T, Kishi S. Progressive enlargement of scattered photocoagulation scars in diabetic retinopathy. Retina 2004;24:507-11.

3.   Browning DJ, Fraser CM. The predictive value of patient and eye characteristics on the course of subclinical diabetic macular edema. Am J Ophthalmol 2008;145:149-154.

Schatz H, Madeira D, McDonald HR, Johnson RN. Progressive enlargement of laser scars following grid laser photocoagulation for diffuse diabetic macular edema. Arch Ophthalmol 1991;109:1549-51.

Treatment techniques and clinical guidelines for photocoagulation of diabetic macular edema. Early Treatment Diabetic Retinopathy Study Report Number 2. Early Treatment Diabetic Retinopathy Study Research Group. Ophthalmology 1987;94:761-74.

Chew EY, Ferris FL III. Nonproliferative Diabetic Retinopathy. In: Ryan SJ. Retina, 4th ed. Philadelphia: Elsevier Mosby, 2006:v.2, pp 1271-1284.

Folk JC, Pulido JS. Laser photocoagulation of the retina and choroid. San Francisco: American Academy of Ophthalmology, 1997.

Basic and Clinical Science Course Section 12: Retina and Vitreous. San Francisco: American Academy of Ophthalmology, 2008: pp 109-132

Bressler NM, Ahmed IIK. Essential OCT. Dublin: Carl Zeiss Meditech, 2006.

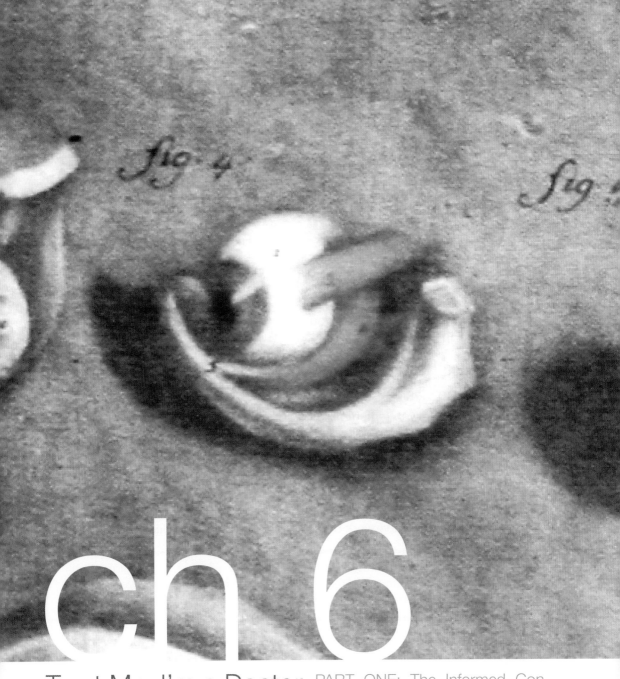

ch 6

Trust Me, I'm a Doctor
PART ONE: The Informed Consent for Treating Diabetic Macular Edema.

THE INFORMED CONSENT for Treating DME

Patient communication is extremely important when one uses lasers to treat diabetic retinopathy. You must remember that in spite of your best efforts to relate the concepts involved, there is a strong tendency for the patient's expectations to be very different from reality. It is certainly reasonable to provide the patient with ancillary information, such as discussions with office staff, video tapes, and handouts. But don't depend on such things to replace you. (Besides, when was the last time you read that handout your dentist gave you about proper flossing?) Ultimately, it is the relationship that you foster with the patient that will—hopefully—keep them motivated to persist with the generally distasteful and often-lifelong pursuit of having their retinas lasered.

You should, first of all, take a deep breath and try not to display the overwhelming sense of near-drowning that one feels on a busy clinic day. You don't necessarily need to slow down so much that you can light your corncob pipe and wax nostalgic about doing lasers with Laura Ingalls Wilder at the Little House on the Prairie. You should, however, remember that your patient will not be impressed by how many exams and lasers you can cram into an hour, but rather, by whether you take the time to carefully explain things, answer questions and skillfully anticipate unvoiced concerns. Make sure there is a family member or friend in the room, too. Having another person in the room will give the patient someone to share the experience with, and the second set of ears will be more functional than those of a stressed-out patient. It is simply a given that the average patient will be unlikely to remember much of what you say. Priluck, et al., wrote a fascinating paper on the ability of patients to recall an informed consent discussion concerning retinal detachment surgery.[1] On average, patients could only remember about 57% of what they had been told, and only 23% remembered the discussion of surgical risks.* Furthermore, patients would commonly state that anything that they did not remember had not been discussed. This is why you have to hyper-document anything you say—because in the polemic world of legal medicine, the paperwork becomes the reality, which is kind of absurd.

> *And only 3% remembered that they could have a hemorrhage or infection that could destroy the eye. Think about *that* the next time you give some wired boomer attorney your best clear-lens-extraction spiel.

What all this really means, though, is that if you truly care more about your patients than about how your paperwork might look to a trial lawyer, you should realize that the data you provide may not be as important as the way in which you deliver it. A machine gun burst of risks will get the job done fast and will meet the "letter of the law" in your chart, but it is unlikely that the patient will remember much of it. However, a slow, careful discussion, with attention to the patient's concerns, will create a far better memory of the mood of the process in the patient's mind, even if the actual facts can't be remembered. Simply knowing that the doctor is actually *interested* in trying to transmit the information may be as important as how much is retained. In other words, you can probably deliver an informed consent in a completely unintelligible language, like maybe Klingon, but if you do it in a way that conveys that you will take all the time in the world to be sure the patient understands the situation, you will have accomplished a lot more than if you list the complications and then have them sign on the dotted line. (That was perhaps a bit hyperbolic, but hopefully the point is made.)

> **On a darker note,** remember that although you know you are a good person, people are constantly reading articles about maniac doctors cutting off the wrong leg or defrauding Medicare. In addition to having trouble understanding the nature of diabetic retinopathy in general, patients may also have an imperceptible lack of trust that can blossom into something really bad if a complication occurs. You have to anticipate this and recognize that careful communication from the start is the best way to avoid trouble.

In any event, here are the concepts to convey, regardless of how you choose to convey them (preferably *not* in Klingon)...

THE DISEASE

You have to make sure the patient has at least a rudimentary understanding of the pathophysiology involved by using your favorite analogy. For diabetic macular edema, this usually involves something like, "the diabetes has changed the blood vessels in your eye from nice new pipes into old rusty pipes, and they are leaking the clear fluid that is in blood. This makes the retina swell up like a tiny sponge in the same way the old veins in people's legs can leak and let their ankles swell up." Or anything similar to that—you can adjust it to the patient's level of interest and sophistication.

It is important to point out that, with macular edema, the vessels are not hemorrhaging actively; many times patients will have been told that they have "burst blood vessels" or "hemorrhages in their eyes," and they visualize some horrible Niagara Falls of blood exploding out of their head. Terms like this generate unnecessary stress, and patients will wonder why you aren't treating the whole thing as a dire emergency and immediately lasering their gushing blood vessels into submission. You really want to dwell on the fact that you are dealing with interstitial fluid leakage and that any microscopic blood spots are really just old bruising and not any sort of active hemorrhage. Incidentally, using the word "bruising" to refer to intraretinal hemorrhages of any sort seems to be a much less inflammatory term than "blood" or "hemorrhage." It tends to avoid the whole Quentin-Tarantino-*Kill-Bill* connotation and gives you a fighting chance that the patient's mind will not seize up and will, instead, continue to follow your discussion.

It is extremely useful to have the patient's photographs, fluorescein angiogram and/or OCT available to show them during this discussion. If you can demonstrate a normal-looking fundus and then show them their own hard exudates and blot hemorrhages moving into the fovea, it is a lot easier for them to understand the gravity of this situation, especially if they do not have a lot of symptoms. This also allows you to point out the fact that you are treating well away from the center of the vision. You would be surprised at how many patients have an unvoiced concern that your main goal is to simply chop away at their vision like a Civil War barber-surgeon and that, just maybe, they might be better off going blind slowly without treatment, rather than letting you hurry things along with your foolish laser.

THE GOALS OF TREATMENT

The patient must also understand the goals of the treatment. They strongly assume that your laser will help improve things. Partly, this is because any time they have gone to a doctor in the past, the doctor usually does something that makes their life better, such as fix a sore throat or stitch a cut. They also know lots of people who have had lasers (YAG and LASIK) and who saw much better immediately after the laser; the distinction between your laser and those lasers can be quite, uh, blurry.

Welcome to the world of retina—a place where patients tend to get worse no matter what you do, and where you will spend a ton of time trying to convince your patients (and perhaps yourself) that going bad slowly is the greatest thing on the planet.

You need to clearly point out that without treatment there is a very good chance the patient will be losing vision over the next one to two years, and that the goal of treatment is to slow down the rate of decay so that instead of ending up terrible, they end up only a little bit worse. This concept is remarkably hard to convey to even a sophisticated patient. Many doctors use terms that suggest to the patient that their vision will stabilize, but even in the best of circumstances, most diabetics don't remain the same.

Here is why you can't promise them stability: Even if your laser works superbly, diabetics can still have gradual deterioration of their visual quality—the fine print is harder to read, going from light to dark is trickier, it is harder to see traffic signs, etc. Although you can very effectively overcome large-scale damage like macular edema, you cannot as easily overcome the gradual deterioration of retinal function that occurs at the cellular level with diabetes. And, as with many retinal treatments, you may be very happy with the results but the patients usually aren't, and they will be particularly unhappy if you have not made sure that they have appropriate expectations.

You may also find that this discussion needs to be repeated at every visit, which becomes tedious, but the perception that diabetics have of the laser can change over time. Initially, there is a strong tendency for patients to assume that a given treatment will make them better, and you have to address such expectations as discussed above. Later on, there is a tendency to assume that any visual problems they have must be from the laser and not from progression of their disease, and you often have to constantly address this as well. Don't forget that you devoted a large chunk of your life to understanding the statistics that make your treatment logical, but these concepts are very new and counterintuitive to your patients.

The best way to understand this is to go back to the graph in Chapter 5 that shows the ETDRS results for treating macular edema. From the standpoint of a treating physician, the graph is great, but Figure 1 shows what it looks like if it is flipped around so you see it from the standpoint of a patient. Although everyone can agree that the control group did horribly, it is clear that, even with treatment, there is a downward trend—especially if the patient lives for any length of time. You might even consider giving patients a crash course in Cartesian coordinates by using your hand to display a rapid downhill course without treatment and then a gentle downhill course with treatment in order to help them understand what they may expect.

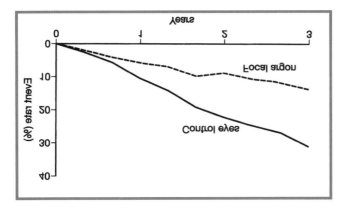

Figure 1. A "patient's eye" view of the graph from Chapter 5 showing the ETDRS results for treating macular edema. This graph makes doctors happy, but this view shows the need to constantly remind the patient about having realistic expectations; diabetic eye damage can still drag the patient downhill, even with perfect treatment. Note the elegant symbolism suggested by the flipped labels: The doctor has to totally wrap his or her head around the patient's point of view to really be able to relate. This was not done because it is easier to flip the original image without changing the labels—it was done on purpose for art's sake.

Of course, patients *can* improve, or at least stabilize, especially with good control and careful laser (and judicious use of intraocular medications if needed—see Chapter 11). They are no longer condemned to follow the dotted line in the graph above. The problem is that if you dwell too much on the possibility of stability or improvement, it may be all the patient remembers of your discussion. They can then become very frustrated with the reality of treatment and end up not returning for follow up. This is by far the worst possible outcome, because they usually return only when they have severe symptoms and awful disease that may be impossible to control. You must anticipate and address anything that may interfere with compliance from the beginning. (See the section at the end of the chapter about treating retinopathy in developing countries for an expanded explanation of this.)

Don't forget that there is another big reason why a patient may want to blame your laser for vision problems, even if the treatment is working perfectly: It is reassuring for some patients to be able to blame the treatment because it is a lot easier to do that than to accept the responsibility for years of poor control. The only way you can work around this is with continual education—and sometimes you have to accept the fact that you will always be the bad guy, even if you have snatched such a patient from the jaws of blindness.

There is one big problem, though, with trying to convey the reality of treating diabetic retinopathy. It turns out that if you communicate this information effectively, and if patients seem to understand the possible "slower rate of decay" concept, they may then draw an additional conclusion that is very erroneous (and you may not hear about it). They may well assume that you mean that they will go downhill forever and that, at best, you will only slow down their inevitable descent into total blindness.

Anticipate this type of conclusion as well, and try to head it off. Remind them that although you can never guarantee anything, it is very unlikely that they will go totally blind from diabetic macular edema, especially if they are good about their control and follow up. Explain that, over time, they may be irritated by their vision, but they are unlikely to ever become helpless, which is what they really fear. Again, throw in plenty of "no guarantees" so their conclusion pendulum doesn't swing to the other side and have them thinking they are off scot-free— but by giving them this reasonable assurance you may save them lots of unnecessary anxiety.

Have you ever had a patient tell you that some doctor told them that they were going blind when they weren't even close to going blind? You may get a sense of superiority from such a comment—you can reassure the patient (and yourself) that there is no way you would ever be so stupid as to say such a thing. Well, it is hard to imagine that *any* doctor would be so stupid as to say such a thing, but now you can see how a patient could come to such a conclusion after a thorough informed consent.

If you think you are a great communicator and that no patient would ever think that you would say that they are going to go blind, just try this simple experiment: After you explain the potential downhill trend inherent in even successfully treated diabetic retinopathy, ask the patient if this means that they will inevitably go blind. You will be surprised at the answers you get. And get ready to take a deep breath and start over—patience is your most valuable surgical tool.

COMPLICATIONS

This is tricky. Never underestimate a patient's ability to mentally assign a huge significance to a tiny risk of complications while ignoring the vastly greater risk of vision loss if they do not get treated. This is especially important to remember in the setting of diabetic retinopathy where—once again—even perfect treatment can't always stop the disease. Patients are very likely to remember your discussion of complications as their vision gets a bit blurrier over time and then they can assume the laser is the problem, even if the blurriness has nothing to do with any laser complication. This puts them on the path to the Dark Side of Noncompliance—something to be avoided if at all possible. The point is that you have to cover the bad things but think carefully about how you do it.

You will be a sucky doctor if you do not make sure patients hear the words "There is a small chance that the laser can make you worse." Even if you become a laser sensei, it is a sad medical fact that bad things can happen, and you never know when both you and the patient will get an unpleasant surprise. You do not want any patient coming back at you claiming that you never said such a thing—no matter how bullet-proof your malpractice carrier says your written informed consent is.

However, you should not leave this (or any other negative concept) hanging at the end of a conversational paragraph. You need to remind them in the following sentence that the risk of treatment is very tiny, but the risk of permanent loss of vision is extremely large without treatment.

Another important warning should be mentioned, especially for Astute Patients (i.e., engineering types): Sometimes, a good observer may forever-after identify the laser spots that you placed in their paramacular vision. This is surprisingly unlikely—most patients are really oblivious of careful, gentle laser for macular edema. However, some patients will notice this, and you get lots of style points for mentioning it before they come to you to complain about it. The key "next-sentence" point to make, though, is that this problem is rare, and even if they do notice something, it is a heck of a lot better to have a few spots on one's peripheral vision than to lose chunks of central vision from untreated disease.

Okay. Once you have gotten the part about the laser making things worse out of the way, it is now even more important to dwell on the biggest problem with the laser: that it may not completely control the disease. Some of this has to do with the general tendency of diabetics to have slowly degraded vision just from being diabetic, as was discussed in the preceding paragraphs. Patients also need to understand that areas of leakage may develop rapidly in any location the diabetes chooses, and even if the treatment works well in one area, the vision may deteriorate if new leaks continue to show up. Patients must be prepared for the possibility of multiple treatments and rapid worsening of vision from progressive disease.

Then you can add that, unfortunately, there are times when the treatment simply does not work at all, and some patients go downhill even with treatment. You can then allude to more aggressive and risky treatments, such as intravitreal steroids, that may help them if the laser can't. Don't let them feel that these more aggressive treatments are Good Things, though. It is easy for patients to think, "Oh well, if the laser doesn't work I'll just have an injection or two and be fine." They need to know that it is much better if they can be controlled with safer, simpler things like a gentle focal laser—in other words, that there is not necessarily a pot of gold at the end of your coherent light rainbow. This is also a good time to emphasize the importance of good systemic control so the patient understands that the laser alone is not going to solve their problem—the patient needs to be an active participant in this process. (Much more on this in The Chapter with a Tantalizing Name.)

As you read this, it may seem like a lot of information to convey when time is limited. However, it really just takes about five minutes to go through this—including the time it takes to be sure patients clearly understand the goals of the treatment. Indeed, making sure the patient understands is perhaps the most important part. The best way to do this is simply to ask patients in a non-judg-mental way to repeat the gist of what you have said and then review any areas that aren't clear. Again, the actual treatment will soon become the least of your worries; making sure that patients understand what you are doing is a job that never stops.

Special Problems with Informed Consent in Developing Countries
(and uniquely American institutions such as free clinics, county hospitals, and other examples of how the American healthcare system can bring third-world medicine to your backyard)

The bulk of this chapter refers to dealing with patients who have a fighting chance of taking good care of themselves. It is also hoped this book will be helpful in situations where patients have less of an opportunity to obtain state-of-the-art healthcare—and the extended section title will hopefully remind read-ers in a certain developed country without universal coverage to keep on read-ing, because there are special problems that arise when resources are limited, no matter what the gross domestic product happens to be.

Developing regions are cursed with a combination of limited healthcare re-sources and a limited desire on the part of the diabetic population to access healthcare until their disease is far advanced. The reasons for the latter are nu-merous and include the cost, the difficulty of obtaining an exam, and the lack of symptoms until things are really bad. One big problem is the perennial dilemma inherent in treating diabetic retinopathy: the perception, on the part of patients, that laser treatment causes blindness.

This dilemma deserves further elaboration. Cataract surgery in developing countries (or any country, for that matter) is met with enthusiasm because the patients experience immediate benefit, and once a cataract is popped out, the problem tends to be over. This sets a level of expectation that is never met by treating diabetic retinopathy in the same setting. Treating diabetic retinopathy usually involves recurring, unpleasant treatments, and there is usually no benefit that the patient can perceive.

This is because diabetics in this situation tend to seek evaluation only when they are forced to by progressive symptoms, at which point their disease is very advanced. Laser treatment is then attempted, and although the treatment usually helps somewhat, the patients still develop severe vision loss. Although one can explain this course of events to patients and their families, there is an inevitable tendency for patients to assume that the laser was the cause of their disease progression rather than to understand that their disease was so hopelessly advanced that the laser could only partially slow the process. The problem is exacerbated by the fact that the affected population tends to be unsophisticated and to have a hard time understanding the nuances discussed in this chapter. The problem is even further exacerbated by the fact that the healthcare workers have limited time and resources to convey such nuances—let alone have time or equipment to perform the treatments.

A vicious circle is then created as patients receive treatment and then go out and tell their friends and family that the laser is "bad." The word spreads, and then more diabetics become afraid to come in for early screening and treatment, and then these diabetics show up with advanced disease that the laser can't stop, and then they think the laser is "bad" because they became worse, and then they tell their friends, and so on and so forth. The problem is compounded by extremely poor systemic control, which makes even timely treatment much less effective.

Overcoming these obstacles by improving the education, monitoring and treatment of diabetics is way outside the scope of this book (although screening with cheap, portable retinal cameras using non-ophthalmic personnel is one way to start). What is well within the scope of this book is how this type of situation can change how the informed consent is presented to the patient. When these patients come crashing into the system with horrible disease, you have to be a bit more blunt and you have to try to offset the whole "laser is bad" thing right from the start. You have to lay out the above facts so the patient understands that your goal is to try to hold on to any vision whatsoever and that they cannot expect to get better or even remain stable. Emphasize that you are going to do everything you can to help them, and it will be a heck of a lot better than doing nothing, but things would have been a lot better if you had seen them well before this point.

You can also beat on them about control, but there may not be much they can do about it in their circumstances. What is really important is that you beat on them to be sure their relatives get checked for diabetes regularly, and if they are found to have diabetes, then they *have* to get an eye exam once a year. Also, if the patient knows anyone with diabetes, they should tell that person to get in for regular eye exams—no matter what—because if that person doesn't, they may end up in the same mess that the patient is facing.

All this sounds harsh, but you really have to go after the tendency for folks to expect that diabetic lasers will solve their visual problems in this situation *and* you have to try to break the vicious cycle of having patients being unwilling or afraid to get an exam and then showing up too late. Finally, you have to try to do all this in a setting where your time and resources are likely very limited.

If you are in such a situation—ask for help. There are international organizations that may be able to lend a hand. The American Academy of Ophthalmology maintains a list of such organizations on their web site (http://www.aao.org/international/links.cfm). There may also be local religious or service-group organizations that can help you—ask around and contact as many people as you can. You may be very surprised at what a difference you can make for your practice and your patients if you are persistent. You are also welcome to write to the address in the introduction—just try not to get frustrated and give up.

Finally, there will be sections in the upcoming chapters that address how one needs to alter the treatment approach in locations where resources are limited and patients with awful disease are plentiful. It turns out that the focus of the informed consent is not the only thing that may be very different these situations.

References and Suggested Reading

1.   Priluck IA, Robertson DM, Buettner H. What patients recall of the preoperative discussion after retinal detachment surgery. Am J Ophthalmol 1979;87:620-3.

Morgan LW, Schwab IR. Informed consent in senile cataract extraction. Arch Ophthalmol 1986;104:42-5.

Herz DA, Looman JE, Lewis SK. Informed consent: is it a myth? Neurosurgery 1992;30:453-8.

VanNewkirk, M. ed. International Ophthalmology. San Francisco: American Academy of Ophthalmology, 2005.

Schwab, L. Eye Care in Developing Nations, 4th Ed. Manson Publishing, 2007.

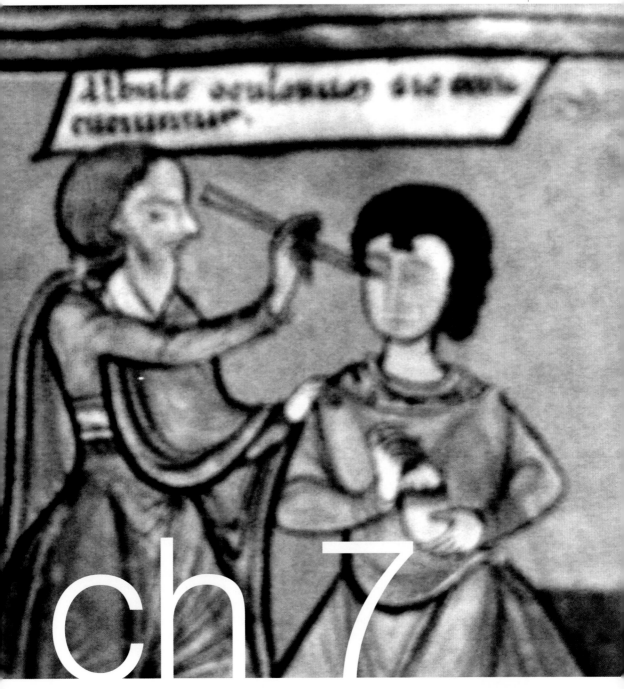

ch 7

Actually Doing a Laser for Macular Edema

GETTING THINGS LINED UP at the Laser

First of all, the patient should be as comfortable as possible under the circum-stances. One of the best ways to facilitate this is to allow someone else to stuff a diagnostic contact lens onto your eye at some point during your training. As you experience this, try to study their every move and your response to each move. Based on how it feels you will develop nuances that will allow you to be much gentler with your patients.

The slit lamp table should be at a comfortable height, and check that the patient is not straining to be in position without realizing it because they are nervous and trying to not be a nuisance. Handles on the table are extremely useful—it gives them something to hold on to and steady their torso. Also, make sure their legs are comfortable, even if you have to straddle their feet.

Make sure that you talk the patient through the entire process. Try to proceed slowly and explain each maneuver prior to doing it. There are books written on how to almost hypnotize the patient with a calm, mantra-like repetition of phras-es. You can get as new-age as you want, but the important thing is to always tell a patient what you are going to do before you do it.

Remember that for many patients the primary association they have with lasers is the image of the planet Alderaan exploding in the first Star Wars movie. Reas-sure them that you are using microscopic powers on your laser and that as long as they are reasonably cooperative, they simply cannot make a mistake. This will relieve them of any fear that they may have about having the success of the treatment rest solely on their shoulders—let them know that it does not make any difference if they blink or sneeze and that you are certainly not going to blow their head off no matter what they do.

> **There is one other thing to discuss,** especially if this is their first laser. You need to warn them that when the laser is over, their vision will be essentially black and their eye will feel glued shut. The laser is so bright that most pa-tients see almost nothing for a few minutes, and the methylcellulose makes them feel like their eye is full of paste. These are really important things to mention. You can lay out the most masterful informed consent, but if you have not prepared the patient for this particular moment, you may have a very upset patient. This is particularly true if you have just treated a one-eyed patient. Fortunately, the darkness fades quickly and then they will see the world in shades that are opposite the wavelength of your laser—usually red if you have a green laser. Patients can easily deal with this as long as you let them know about it in advance.

Unless they are laser veterans, they will still be rather anxious at this point. Perhaps the most useless phrase in the world is "try to relax." Nothing can whip a patient into a frenzy faster than an instruction like this. It is much better to offer specific suggestions. For instance, as the patient leans forward to the slit lamp, you may want to put your hand on their neck and shoulder to both guide them and to see how tight their trapezius is. Because it is always as taut as a guitar string, you can tell them to try to relax their neck and shoulders and let the chin rest do the work of holding their head up. By focusing on a specific task, they can have more of a definite goal than just "relax."

The same is true for the inevitable battle with the contact lens. If you tell them to hold still and try not to blink you might as well inject them with pure meth-amphetamine and see whether they can shake your slit lamp right off the table. Instead, you may want to consider telling them to blink as much as they want, but to also concentrate on keeping their forehead pressed against the bar. This way, they can focus on just this rather simple task, which is far more useful to you than yearning for some fairyland where patients actually open their eyes and stop blinking when you ask them to.

Figure 1 demonstrates a reasonable way to work with recalcitrant eyelids. It is useful if the patient can look down; this allows you to place your thumb over the tarsal plate, which gives you a lot of control over the upper lid. At the same time, you can use the ring finger of the other hand to pull the lower lid down while keeping the contact lens between the thumb and first two fingers. If the patient is truly concentrating on keeping their forehead against the bar, you will be able to generate an effective amount of static friction on the eyelids, and then you can easily separate the lids and get the contact lens inserted. This is where a small flange on the lens is extremely useful, because once you have control of the upper lid and the flange is behind the lower lid, the lens will almost insert itself. Also, with a good flange, the patient will be unable to squeeze the lens out even if they could crush a Volkswagen with their orbicularis. The bigger the flange, the more secure the lens; but there is a balance, because as the flange gets bigger it is harder to get the lens in.

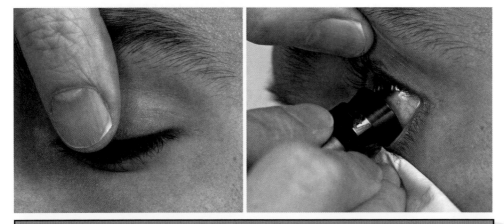

Figure 1. The left photo shows how you can have the patient look down, allowing you to put your thumb in contact with the entire width of their tarsal plate. This gives you maximum traction to pull the lid up and get it out of the way. You can then have them look up in order to make the lower lid more lax and make the patient less likely to see the lens coming. You can then pull the lower lid down with the side of your ring finger, hook the flange over the lower lid, and rotate the lens into the eye. In this case, a tissue is folded up and held between the ring and little fingers to help with traction and to catch any contact lens gel that oozes out of the eye. You want to do this because the gel can run down next to the nose and drive patients nuts during the treatment. (Photos by James Whitcraft, IPFW)

If the eyelids don't get out of the way, you will have an excellent magnified view of their eyelashes at this point. Occasionally you can rescue this situation by having them look in the direction of the eyelid that is under the flange and pushing the lens in the direction of the lid that is properly placed in front of the flange. If the lids are loose enough, you can pull the offending eyelid back over the flange. Most of the time, however, the whole region has been turned into a slippery mess by the contact lens gel, and you have to bail out and start all over again. Make sure you do a Zen breath and wall off any bubbling frustration—patients can detect your irritation with remarkable sensitivity and they will then go into a positive-feedback loop of increasing anxiety and lock their eye shut.

> **Incidentally,** when you first put the methylcellulose on the lens it helps to squeeze it first onto a tissue, rather than onto the lens. The first drop often has little bubbles that have a sentient ability to get in your way when you do the laser.

If you are truly unable to get the lens in you can do a lid block as a last resort, but if you have to do this more than once or twice in your career, you may want to re-assess how you insert contact lenses—the problem may lie with someone other than the patient. If you are self-aware enough to wonder whether your technique is suboptimal, the best way to find out for sure is to try putting a laser lens on your spouse. Seriously. They will be more than happy to let you know how you are doing it wrong—that is why you married them in the first place.

In any event, once you finally get the lens in place, you should take a moment to congratulate yourself; you have overcome approximately 50 years million years of evolution and actually convinced a stranger to let you shove something into their eye. You should also take a moment to make sure the patient hasn't shifted out of the ideal position in the slit lamp—they can twist out of position, which can make doing the laser very difficult. Which leads us to the next potential problem.

FIXATION

Getting the patient to look in the right direction can be a daunting task. You will rapidly learn that some patients are utterly precise in their ability to fixate on the target light, and you will thereby learn the art of nailing microaneurysms with barely a whisper of RPE change. Most patients are reasonably accurate, so you can get the job done with minimal fuss. There are occasional patients, however, who make you feel like you are trying to split a diamond during a dune buggy ride, and it is for these that the following section exists.

As with telling them to relax, you have probably figured out that the worst thing you can do is to demand that the patient hold still and stare at the frickin' fixation light. So try a bit of the old word massage: Keep a soothing stream of chatter going—what you say is not as important as how you say it. You can let them know how well they are doing and how well the treatment is going as you chase their perifoveal retina all over the place. (Relax; there was a Papal bull in 1674 saying it is OK to lie to patients while doing a laser.) You can point out that the treatment you are about to apply is so delicate that they wouldn't feel it on their skin, and that everything will be okay if they end up blinking or sneezing or whatever because you can stop anytime. This warm fuzzy stuff does not always work with a fidgety patient, but it provides a good mantra to help you keep your cool.

Other options to encourage fixation include:

1. Sometimes they do not realize that their fixating eye is closed—a gentle reminder will help them realize this, and it may solve the problem.

2. The above is usually too easy; they can't open their eye because they are nervously squeezing both eyes shut. If they can't keep their fixating eye open, then bail out and encourage them keep their fixating eye closed. Sometimes this will get them to relax enough so that even if they aren't quite staring in the right direction, they at least won't be moving all over the place—that is, they won't be futilely struggling with themselves to force their eye open when they simply can't do it. The eye you are working on may Bell up, so you will probably have to shove the lens superiorly to get a better view. Occasionally, patients will have a tendency to look in some weird direction like far right or left when their eyes are closed, so if your view doesn't improve when you push up on the lens, you should lift the eyelid over the "fixating" eye to find out where it is looking. By the way, this is where it is really important to be able to use an indirect contact lens as discussed in Chapter 4—such lenses are much less dependent on patient cooperation and your fixation blues will largely disappear.

3. If your lens has a large flange, you can also try pushing relatively hard on the eye to keep it steady, although sometimes the discomfort makes things worse. As in vasovagal worse. Careful with this one, especially in younger male patients.

4. You can treat all the lesions that are relatively far away from the fovea first. You have to be sure you don't lose your landmarks and accidentally work your way into fovea-land, but sometimes the constant dazzle to these less critical areas will desensitize the patient, so by the time you work your way closer to the center, things are not as jumpy.

5. You can default to a total grid mode and give up on true focal treatment—simply get in spots as safely as you can around the thickened areas. This is somewhat less than optimal, especially if there is a lot of focal disease, but it is better than nothing.

6. Finally, there are some patients who simply need a retrobulbar block to gain control of the situation. You will probably want to consider this sooner, rather than later, in a patient who has clear-cut focal disease but will not hold still. As will be discussed in the next chapter, a carefully applied focal treatment may reverse things tremendously with only minimal changes at the level of the RPE. A shotgun grid performed in desperation on a moving target may chew up a lot of valuable retina that the patient might prefer to have around for the rest of their life. Under these circumstances, it is probably safer to use a block and do a proper focal than to get frustrated and do a suboptimal grid treatment. Always remember the risk-benefit ratio of an office block, though. The phrase "this is your brain on drugs" takes on a whole new meaning if you squirt lidocaine into someone's brainstem (more on this in Chapter 15).

> **Some experts recommend** using an oral anxiolytic. There are some patients that do prefer some type of sedation, but it is a lot of hassle for a few minutes of laser time. Also, these drugs are often not strong enough to make a difference unless you go for anesthetic doses, which is not a good idea in a laser room. Occasional patients may benefit, though, so don't forget that you were once a real doctor and that you do have this option.

What if they have too much fixation?

The yin to the yang of poor fixation is the tendency for patients to stare directly at your slit lamp light and thereby put the aiming beam right on their fovea at all times. You need to tell them to avoid this, but do so gently, and recognize once again that repetition of this instruction rapidly becomes counterproductive, especially if the pitch of your voice gets higher and higher. Better to tell them once, and then mildly suggest that they imagine they are looking off into the distance while you start treating well away from the fovea to desensitize them, as mentioned above. You have to be really careful as you move closer to the foveal area, because these patients may suddenly swing right into the light—so have a light foot on the trigger. This type of patient can be way more stressful than the patient with poor fixation, because you never know when they might shift their fovea onto your metaphorical hand grenade.

OK, several pages and a couple thousand words and we have just reached the point where you can start lasering. Read on...

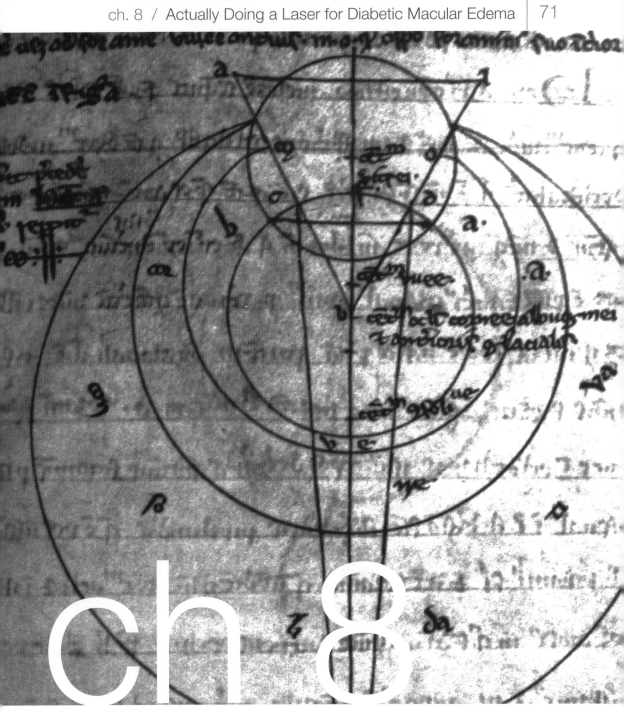

ch 8

The Chapter That is Really About Actually Doing a Laser for Diabetic Macular Edema

If you paid attention to the last chapter you are about ready to start lasering. If you didn't read the last chapter then your surgical pyramid may be on shaky ground— you have to unconsciously be doing everything in Chapter 7 in order to have a fighting chance of actually doing the good stuff in Chapter 8. And here it is…

SPOT POWER and a Little About Spot Size

There are a number of different approaches to the laser treatment for diabetic macular edema. The traditional ETDRS approach was to start with a 50-micron spot and .1-second duration. Then treatment was initiated with a power of 50 milliwatts, and this was gradually increased in 10- to 20-mW increments until a color change occurred in the offending microaneurysm. (This direct treatment of a microaneurysm is referred to as focal treatment.) If there was diffuse leakage without any obvious focal source, then grid treatment was applied, consisting of light burns of 50 to 100 microns spaced >1 burn width apart.

> **For this discussion** it is assumed you are using a duration of .1 second, although as long as you are careful with the other parameters it does not make that much difference—most doctors use something between .05 to .2 seconds. The longer durations use lower powers to get the same effect so the burn builds up slowly and can be titrated easily (recall the energy density equation in Chapter 3). On the other hand, a longer burn gives the patient more time to move and mess up your shot. Shorter durations need more power but some doctors prefer to obtain a quick hit that is relatively independent of patient movement. However, you have to be very careful to avoid a rapid buildup of the burn given the small spot and the higher power, especially given the variable pigmentation and retinal thickness that can be present in the macula.

Depending on the laser and the eye, you will usually start getting some sort of uptake around 80 to 110 mW, although the actual power requirements may vary a great deal depending on the thickness of the retina, media opacity and fundus pigmentation. For instance, black or Hispanic patients with clear media may need very little power, perhaps as little as 60 to 70 mW. Paler fundi may need frighteningly large powers, especially if there is any sort of cataract or grubby capsule. Clean pseudophakia, on the other hand, can let you get a hot burn very easily, whatever the pigmentation—be very careful and start with a very low power, especially if you have been learning your trade by treating through typical diabetic nuclear and cortical opacities.

Exactly what kind of burn are you looking for? No one knows. Even though the ETDRS called for "light" burns, you can see from Figure 1 that they could still be fairly white and hot (Figure 1 is from a teaching series from the 1980s). There are those who feel that if you want ETDRS results, you have to treat like the ETDRS, but most folks nowadays think "less is more" and will use much lighter burns.

Here are just a few reasons why: First of all, Figure 2 reminds you that the spots you put in are like gifts that keep on giving—they can slowly enlarge long after you have moved on. Second, it makes sense to treat with milder burns—simply because you can always go back and apply more treatment, but you cannot undo overly aggressive treatment. Finally, diabetics live a lot longer than they did back when the ETDRS was performed, and they tend to have better control. Better control means that they will respond better to milder treatment, and a longer life means that there is more time for any spots you put in to expand.

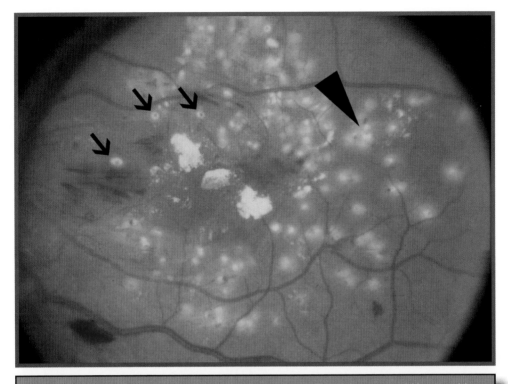

Figure 1. This is a training slide from over 25 years ago. These burns would be considered a bit hot nowadays, although one could argue that this eye is in trouble and should be hit hard (note the hard exudates building up in the fovea). Also note the extremely satisfying bombs dropped squarely on some of the microaneurysms (arrows). Ideally you would want to use a smaller spot to try and treat only the microaneuysm and minimize collateral damage. Also notice the classic pattern that occurs when the patient moves just enough to keep you from hitting a microaneurysm dead on and you end up peppering the entire area around it in frustration (arrowhead). This shows why you should not keep firing away at a moving target—you can take out a lot of retina with multiple spots trying to get one little microaneurysm. (Courtesy of the Early Treatment Diabetic Retinopathy Research Group)

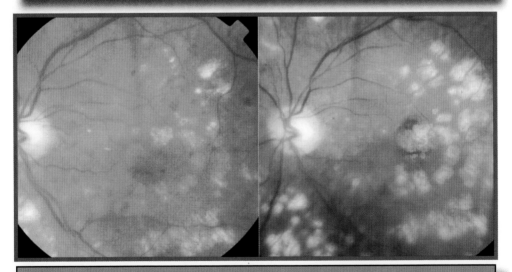

Figure 2. Note enlargement of laser scars—especially the confluence of the scars around the fovea. This is why you need to tread lightly.

Also, diabetic maculas don't tend to fall apart quickly, and you don't need to feel like your first treatment is the only thing standing between your patient and a white cane—especially if the patient has reasonable diabetic control and the disease is away from the fovea.

Practically speaking, this means that the goal is often a very subtle, small burn—something that just begins to show some lightening of the RPE—if you are doing a grid. If there is a lot of diffuse, thick edema, it may be worthwhile to go for a bit more whitening beyond this level, although heavier burns should be done only in areas that are farther from the fovea.

If you are trying to get a specific microaneurysm, the ETDRS wanted you to get some sort of color change within the lesion, either lighter or darker. This is still a nice thing to aim for, but recently there has been more emphasis on just getting the microaneurysm treated and not hammering away until you see a color change.[1] Basically, if you can get a color change, great, but don't go postal trying to get it.

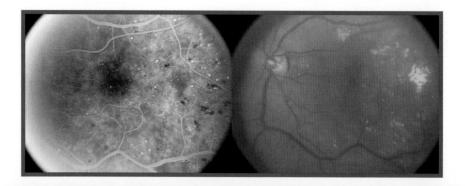

Figure 3. An example of a milder grid. The angiogram shows some microaneurysms but there is also a lot of diffuse leakage in the entire temporal half of the posterior pole. Aggressive white laser spots would create a large scar and likely shove edema right into the fovea. A very light grid can be seen in the area of leakage—this is a good degree of uptake to start with, although in retrospect some of the burns are a bit too close together.

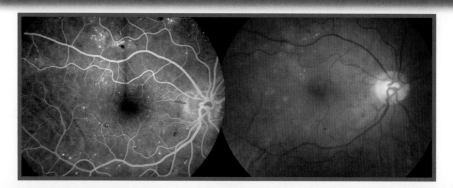

Figure 4. An example of light treatment to areas of focal leakage. These are light burns and if you are worried that they are insufficient you can bring the patient back in six to eight weeks and add more if necessary.

Ultimately, the subtleties of this are learned from clinical experience and not just clinical trials, so understand that these are, at best, guidelines—there is no proven "perfect" burn. Survey the retina people around you and take advantage of any hands-on teaching you can get, and then try to develop a treatment pattern that works best for you. Figures 3 and 4 give examples of milder treatment approaches, and Figure 5 shows the appearance of a mild grid after a number of years.

Whatever burn you are trying for, the first step is to get the tightest focus you can with your aiming beam—if you don't get this first bit right, you will be punching marshmallows and your settings and uptake will be changing all over the place. And don't worry if at first it seems like you are spending hours getting a tight aiming beam and determining an effective power. Review Chapter 7, practice like crazy, and try some of the tricks discussed later in the text. As you develop experience you will be able to rapidly factor in all of the variables and quickly dial in safe and effective settings.

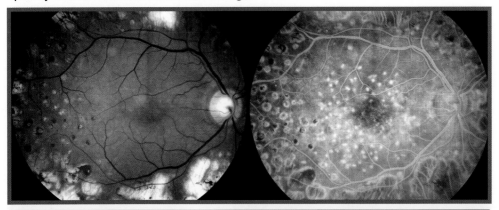

Figure 5. This gives you an idea of how a light grid such as in Figure 4 can look years later. The red free on the left shows that you can barely see the spots that were placed about nine years prior to these photographs. The angiogram on the right lights up the spots. This patient went from 20/200 to 20/60 with laser combined with better systemic control.

SPOT SIZE and a Bit About Spot Power

The main goal is to use the smallest size possible to minimize scar expansion. It is best to start with a 50-micron spot and adjust the power as discussed above (some lasers only go down to 75 microns, which is OK, too). Be warned that 50 (or 75) microns is small, and you need to be very careful that you are not using powers that can accidentally punch through Bruch's membrane.

How do you know if you broke Bruch's? It is usually pretty obvious. First of all, the patient may jump because you will have generated a small popping sound within their head, which is another quick way to lose style points. Also, have you ever been watching a movie when the projector breaks and the heat of the bulb melts the film? The frozen frame gets this weird bubbly look, and then it rapidly melts away from the center, leaving nothing but a blank screen and a faint smell of burning celluloid. This is exactly what a burn in Bruch's membrane is like—but way faster and smaller and hopefully without the smell of something burning. Or at least this is what I have been told. This has, of course, never happened to me. Basically, breaking Bruch's is something that you should only imagine; you should never be using settings that are even close to causing this complication.

The problem is that such a burn is really bad. A hemorrhage may occur and result in immediate loss of vision. (By the way, should there be a hemorrhage, there is something that you should do immediately. Think for a moment about what you would do, because if you end up in this situation, you should be prepared—time is of the essence. If you aren't sure, feel free to do the asterisk thing.*)

A hot burn can also result in the late development of a choroidal neovascular membrane, and you will have given the patient a brand new problem that is way worse than the original disease. By the way, you don't have to break through Bruch's membrane to get a choroidal neovascular membrane to grow—they can occur at any laser spot (although they are more likely with hotter burns closer to the fovea). If a patient starts to get funny-looking pigmentation and edema in a localized area, you need to think about this complication. If you keep treating them with focal laser in a mistaken attempt to treat "diabetic" edema, they will end up with a lot of vision loss that could have been avoided if treated with intra-vitreal therapy (Figure 6).

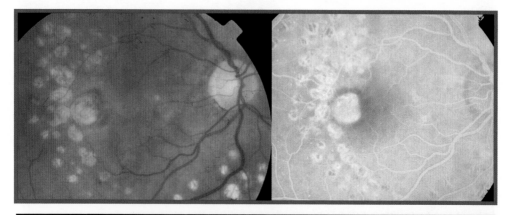

Figure 6. The color shows abnormal pigmentation spreading out from a series of big scars near the fovea. On clinical examination you would see pronounced macular edema in this patient. The FA highlights the presence of a large neovascular membrane growing from the laser scars. This is one of many reasons why you don't want to treat heavily near the fovea.

*Push on the eye like crazy with the contact lens until the bleeding stops! (Warning: This may make some sensitive patients vasovagal—nothing is simple.)

Sometimes, using a 100-micron spot will allow you to laser with "training wheels"—the larger size will keep you from punching through Bruch's membrane, and you do not need a high degree of accuracy if you are trying to get a given microaneurysm. A spot this large uses up a lot of ground in the macula, however. Try to use this size only for more peripheral treatment in order to quickly build up experience—you should use the smallest spot you can, as soon as you can.

There is one technique for focal treatment that uses a two-size approach. First, one places a 100-micron burn at the level of the pigment epithelium beneath the microaneurysm. This white burn will then act as sort of a backstop, because it will not absorb laser energy in the same way that the darker RPE and choroid would. Then you can drop down to a 50-micron spot and treat the microaneurysm more aggressively. (You still have to remember what you are doing to your energy density when you decrease the spot size by this much—backstop or no.*) It is not clear whether this approach is better. In fact, a whole bunch of 100-micron burns around the fovea may be riskier in the long run compared to using 50-micron spots with care. If nothing else, it is good to be aware of techniques like this in order to better know all the tools you have at your disposal.

> *Uh, you do remember this, right? The part of the equation in Chapter 3 that has a tiny "2" in the denominator that means a small change in spot size makes a *big* difference in what you pump into the retina? This concept needs to be so ingrained that if you are captured by aliens and pithed for a science project your decerebrate hands will still reach for the power knob if someone says "smaller spot."

HAVING PICKED OUT a Given Spot Size and a Starting Power...

It is probably best to start somewhere near the inferior arcade, and well away from the fovea, to test the power; patients are less likely to notice anything in the superior visual field if there is a problem. Once you feel you have a reasonably safe power, you can start to work in toward the meaty areas, but remember that variables like foveal pigmentation and retinal thickness may change your laser uptake significantly from your test spots, so proceed carefully.

It is a good idea to pick an unmistakable set of hard exudates, hemorrhages and/or microaneurysms close to the fovea in order to define The Line That You Must Never Cross. As you begin the great video game of focal treatment, it is all too easy to concentrate on the job of shooting at red things and accidentally move into the edge of the foveal avascular zone, particularly if there is a lot of pathology and if the patient is twitchy. Setting up a mental demarcation line around the fovea will make this much less likely—avoiding the fovea should be the focus of your universe for the duration of the treatment. (By the way, try not to let your aiming beam get near the fovea as you study the lay of the land. The odds are you would never accidentally trigger the laser, but there is no need to tempt the gods of retina to teach you a lesson.)

Incidentally, be very careful when treating just below the fovea. Before cutting to the blue box to learn why, take a second to try to figure it out for yourself. Hint:

This is not something to worry about if the patient has been given a retrobulbar anesthetic.

> **Remember Bell's reflex** and how it can change the position of the fundus. If the patient blinks very hard the front of the eye goes up but the back of the eye goes down. If you are treating just below the fovea, the fovea can flip down into your aiming beam faster than your foot can come off the pedal. And that juicy pigment in the fovea will take up laser really fast. Usually you will have a clue that this might happen based on the patient's behavior at the slit lamp and you can be ready to back off immediately if necessary. Also, just to be confusing, you may notice that in some patients the fovea can actually move up with a blink—perhaps as they squeeze they contract multiple extraocular muscles which makes the ocular movement less predictable. Just be careful around the fovea, period.

OK, now you have set your spot size and power, and your mental GPS has set up a barricade around the fovea. You are now ready to cook pathology. The first step is to treat the obvious microaneurysms in a given quadrant. An even first-er step, though, is to figure out which little red spots are really microaneurysms and which are little dot hemorrhages. This is where it is invaluable to have a projected angiogram available when you do these treatments—especially when you are learning.

You will be surprised at how many little red dots in the fundus are not really microaneurysms at all, and you will also be surprised at how many microaneurysms on the angiogram are almost invisible on fundus exam. Some microaneurysms are even a yellowish color and can simulate a small hard exudate. The point is that indiscriminately treating every red spot can result in a lot of unnecessary damage. Furthermore, it is fairly easy to get a blot hemorrhage to change color, and you can incorrectly think you are doing a great job, when really you are just burning up the nerve fiber layer and not treating the actual leaks. Looking carefully at an angiogram as you treat is a great way to understand the pathology—it will help you fine-tune your ability to perceive microaneurysms and help minimize wasted spots from just "shooting red." If you do angiographically guided treatment enough, you will find that you will become much better at both your exam and treatments—and ultimately, you even find that you are less dependent on an angiogram because your clinical exam will be so good. (Figure 7 is a good example of how to approach this—and it is not unique. You will find similar differences between the clinical exam and FA in just about any diabetic if you take the time to look.)

Occasionally, microaneurysms may be yellowed from sclerosis, simulating little chunks of hard exudates, which you would not otherwise treat. The only way to learn about this type of stealth lesion is by studying the angiogram and looking at the patient. If you find one, it means you are ready for your black belt (Figure 8).

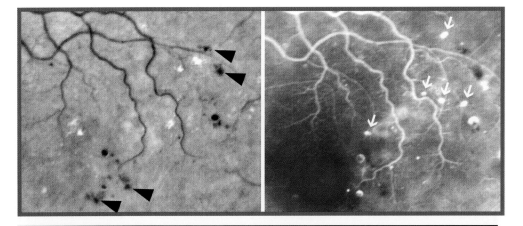

Figure 7. These photos are cool—take some time to study them. First, imagine how you would treat based on the red free photo on the left. Now work through the arrows, comparing the FA to the clinical appearance. The black arrowheads show things that you might have treated as microaneurysms but are really just hemorrhages. Note also that there are at least five troublesome microaneurysms that are essentially invisible on the clinical picture (white arrows). If you were studying the patient with a contact lens you would likely see the corresponding microaneurysms as tiny dots; sometimes you can only see them in the backflash of the laser as you treat in the area. Finally, look at the two obvious microaneurysms next to the foveal avascular zone on both the red free and FA. Although you might be tempted to go after them because they are big and leaky, note that they are part of the few remaining capillaries supplying that side of the fovea. It would be much better to treat everything else first and only go after those two if all else fails—and then go after them very lightly if at all. (Also note the dark center to some of the microaneurysms suggesting that the lumen is partially filled with a clot. This is fairly common in large microaneurysms.)

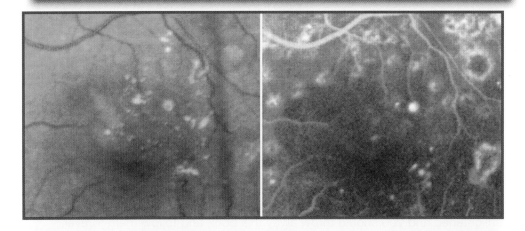

Figure 8. An example of a yellow microaneurysm—in the center of a group of hard exudates. Usually they are not this obvious—they are often much smaller and therefore harder to photograph. They also can be completely yellow; this one has some red showing through the middle. (Extra credit if you can find the other yellowish microaneurysm in the picture.)

Two finesse points:

As you study the patient and the FA you will begin to see that there is a clinically detectable difference between a true microaneurysm and a blot heme "pseudo-microaneurysm." You will get a sense that the real microaneurysms can be seen to be little 3-D spheroid globs, while the hemorrhages are more two-dimensional. This is not always the case, and the lesions need to be on the large size to detect the difference, but it is something to look for.

Another finesse point is to look for tiny microaneurysms in the back scatter of your laser shot. If you think you know where a given microaneurysm might be based on the FA but you really don't see anything clinically then treat the area with a spot. If you look carefully you may be able to see the microaneurysm backlit by the bright coherent laser beam. Obviously one does not randomly treat the retina with laser spots just to find hidden microaneurysms. The point of this is to recognize that information is available to you at all times if you look for it and you may be surprised by what you can see if you study the retinal details that are lit up when you fire the laser.

Having found your targets, it is time for the kill. As mentioned above, the traditional goal is to get the microaneurysm to either darken or lighten, which presumably indicates closure or at least sclerosis of the aneurysm wall (refer to Figure 1). Of course, this represents the Platonic essence of laser treatment perfection. In the shadow world where the rest of us dwell, things are a bit more complicated. First of all, unless the patient is very cooperative, it is often difficult to drill a microaneurysm with this degree of precision—even if you are trying just to hit the microaneurysm without getting a definite color change. Most of the time, the first shot misses to one side and then the second shot misses to the other side, and then you are wondering exactly how many shots you are going to take before you convert the region into a charred landscape while the microaneurysm itself cheerfully stays micro-plump and micro-red while it micro-laughs at you (again, Figure 1).

Take heart—you are not alone. If you ask seasoned retina specialists, you will learn that perhaps only 10 to 20% of all shots end up with a truly satisfying direct hit. Sometimes this percentage can go as high as 80 to 90% if the lesions are discreet and the patient is cooperative. If someone tells you that they routinely hit *all* microaneurysms on *all* patients then they are either (a) a liar; (b) able to alter their reality on some sort of quantum mechanical level so that they aren't technically lying but no one else sees what they are seeing; or (c) they are truly enlightened and you should throw away this book and follow them forever.

In the meantime, we mere mortals are often left in the position of trying to decide what to do once we have used up a few shots and only straddled a given microaneurysm. Discretion is the best part of lasering, and it is probably best to bail out and move on if it looks like you are not making much progress. This is OK, because no one really knows for sure why focal treatment works. Is it changes in the microaneurysm, or is it changes in the retina and retinal pigment epithelium under the microaneurysm? In other words, does the laser work because you are you sealing the leaks with direct hits, or are you helping the RPE to suck out the fluid faster with misses? The effect of laser is probably a combination of these—and no doubt other effects—and that is why you don't have to be anal with those pesky microaneurysms that dodge your laser spots. Practically speaking, if you do want deliver focal treatment and the first couple of shots miss, it is reasonable to move on to the next location, because it is not in your patient's best interest for you to keep hammering away at each microaneurysm until you have a 300-micron treatment and still no direct hit.

> **By the way,** here is something that is fun to do: Go back and look at microaneurysms that you have treated. Even if you do manage to safely achieve the old ETDRS ideal of a change in color, you may find that a number of the treated aneurysms will have reverted back to a reddish color by the time you have finished treating the last of the line. Should you re-treat them? Some will go back and re-treat obvious big ones, but no one knows if this is worth it—whatever you do, don't go crazy over it.

Sometimes there will appear to be a group of microaneurysms heaped up in one area, almost like a cluster of grapes. These areas are usually deceptive, and you should study the angiogram first before leaping in and treating, because you may think that you have the proverbial fish in the barrel. However, if you look carefully at the angiogram, you will see that there are usually only a few real microaneurysms, and the rest of the red dots are just hemorrhages. If you go in and really cook the whole area, you will cause a big burn that usually goes through some of the nerve fiber cables, and you will have been way more aggressive than necessary.

Some patients will have tons of microaneurysms. If this is the case, do not try to treat every single one—you can end up with far-too-confluent treatment because you are dutifully trying to nail every little leak. Rather, treat obvious large ones and try not to put in more than a spot every three to four spot widths apart. It is better to put in some treatment, then wait and add more, rather than to try to treat everything (Figure 9).

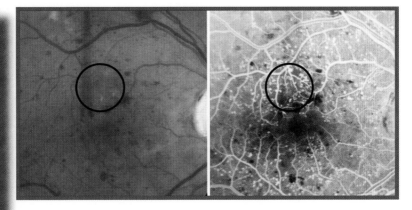

Figure 9. An example of a situation where you do not want to treat every microaneurysm. Aggressive treatment would result in confluent burns—best to go lightly and add more spots over time if necessary. Also note that there are far more microaneurysms on the FA than are apparent clinically. The area in the circle is wall-to-wall microaneurysms but there is almost nothing to see on the color.

Another occasional finding is a really big microaneurysm (maybe 75 to 100 microns—the large yellow one in Figure 8 is an example). These can be really fun, because you can watch them shrivel up nicely as you treat them; but there are a few caveats. First, check the angiogram and make sure the lesion is not part of the only remaining vessel supplying the edge of the fovea. It would be bad to shut down such a vessel. Second, make sure you are not treating a large microaneurysm with a small spot—you can end up puncturing it and making it bleed. Although such a hemorrhage is easy to control, it is still better to carefully increase the spot size and gradually treat the lesion, rather than hitting it with a small, hot burn.

As mentioned above, you do not want to waste time treating small hemorrhages that look like microaneurysms. You also need to take special care when treating near large, obvious hemorrhages. Such hemorrhages will take up the laser dramatically, and you can ruin a lot of the patient's overlying nerve fiber layer. This is particularly dangerous when treating in the papillomacular bundle; a burn here can create a scotoma that is far larger than the size of the original laser spot. This same warning applies if you are re-treating a patient who has old laser scars. The extra pigment will increase uptake and you can cause a bad burn very quickly. (You should be staying away from prior burns in previously treated patients anyway in order to avoid atrophic patches from overlapping treatment.)

> **Another cool thing,** if there is persistent edema, is to repeat an angiogram and look specifically at the microaneurysms that you tried to close with the previous treatment. You may be surprised that these can be frightfully recalcitrant little devils. Note that if you decide to go back and treat the same microaneurysm you need to be careful of the underlying pigment changes caused by the previous laser.

Although it is important not to kill yourself or your patient's RPE in order to nail focal microaneurysms, you should generally make focal treatment your goal as much as possible. First of all, there are few things more satisfying than toasting succulent microaneurysms with a single laser spot that spares the underlying RPE.* The gratification is even greater because, several months later, these patients usually have a marked decrease in their swelling and hard exudates, with little or no evidence of laser treatment. This represents the Holy Grail of focal diabetic treatment, and it is so rewarding that it brings to mind the old learning-psychology axiom, "intermittent reinforcement creates behaviors that are hardest to extinguish." Never extinguish your goal of focal microaneurysm treatment with minimal RPE damage.

Alright, now you have taken out the focal leaks. What if there is a lot of diffuse leakage that doesn't come from obvious microaneurysms? The next step is to perform a light grid to any areas of diffuse leakage, filling in the preexisting focal treatment. Do not get aggressive here—less is definitely way more. *Do not* feel that you have to conquer all the diffuse leakage in one treatment. First of all, many times there are enough microaneurysms that the focal treatment itself cre-

*If you don't think this is satisfying you are a real loser. Get outta here and go do clear lens extractions on patients that think glasses are a disease. Jeez.

ates a sufficient grid. Also, remember that now that the patient is actually being treated for a diabetic complication, he or she may get it through their head that their life and vision depend on taking better care of themselves. This will make a much bigger difference than your laser spots, but it will take a while to pay off. To repeat, patience is your most valuable surgical tool.

If there are areas of thickening that have not been treated by focal laser, then put in a grid pattern using a small spot size with a power that gives you a very light burn. Some folks will increase the spot size as the grid is carried out away from the fovea—ranging from 50 microns near the center, up to 200 microns in the periphery. It may be simpler to just use the same small size and place more spots in the periphery, or to defocus the aiming beam to generate a larger spot (more on the latter technique in the next chapter). Regardless of what you may have read, do not put a lot of spots in the thickened area—and try to avoid placing your burns one spot width apart. Maybe go a nice, wide three or four spot widths apart; you can always add more.

If you need to treat in diffusely thickened retina, there are definitely some things to be aware of. First of all, your beam will diffuse out and you will need to increase the power to get a take. Be *very* careful when you do this—for two reasons:

> 1. If you go back to thinner retina, you can get a really hot burn, which is not a good thing to do near the fovea. (Vide supra about burning celluloid.)

> 2. Even if you use a small spot size, the diffusion of the beam through the thick retina can create a large burn that will come back to haunt you as a giant scar.

Another important thing is to be certain you can remember where you have already done parts of the grid. Light, diffuse burns will fade during the course of your treatment, and you can come back to the same area thinking it hasn't been fully treated. If you decide to add just a bit more laser before you call it a day, you can create confluent lesions without realizing it. The result is way too much treatment that will only be apparent to, for instance, every other doctor who sees the patient for the rest of their life. This is definitely a case where "the enemy of good is perfect." Mentally delineate areas that you have gridded so you don't go back over them repeatedly.

Although the ETDRS used a combination of focal and grid treatment, there is another philosophy that espouses the use of pure grid treatment for everything. This approach applies 100 to 200 micron spots throughout all areas of thickening without necessarily treating specific microaneurysms. A recent study suggested that such an approach—even with much gentler grid treatment—does not seem to be as effective as a focal/grid combination.[1] It is worth mentioning this to point out that although it is easy and tempting to just do a fast grid on everyone, such an approach is neither ideal nor elegant. You should put your shotgun away and concentrate on learning how to treat parsimoniously.

Another thing to keep in mind is that macular edema can actually be exacerbated by overly aggressive treatment. It is natural to want to treat every red spot and swollen area because, well, it is fun to do and you feel you are stamping out blindness. Unfortunately, it is possible to push edema into the fovea with extensive treatment. Patients with fragile vasculature and more diffuse edema are more likely to end up with this problem. It is also more common if there is a "wall" of edema just outside the fovea and you aggressively treat everything in the area of thickening, which can push the wall right into the fovea. You can try to blame this on progression of the patient's underlying disease, rather than a side effect of the laser, and sometimes this will be the case. However, if you really caused the problem there will be no doubt in the patient's mind or in your inner soul that your laser did it—their vision will nosedive and will stay nosedived from the moment you finish the laser.

If you do cause this problem, it will often resolve gradually as your laser reins in the original leakage, but it can take some time. (Good systemic control on the patient's part is helpful here.) You can sit tight and wait, but this is often a good time to get a second opinion to protect yourself and address the patient's understandable concerns. Sometimes these patients will respond nicely to intravitreal therapy as an adjunct to your laser. The key thing to remember is that if you think a patient really requires a lot of macular treatment, you may want to break it up into separate sessions in order to gently get things under control.

But getting back to the treatment…

How far out do you carry your spots? Most people do not treat much beyond the arcades, simply because it is unlikely for there to be any useful effect that far away from the fovea. If there are obvious focal areas of leakage that are trying to stream hard exudates and edema toward the fovea from far away, it certainly makes sense to touch them up. Even if they are far away, it may help decompress more delicate central structures and buy the patient more time. Also, if there is very diffuse thickening beyond the arcades, it may be reasonable to treat further out, simply to preserve peripheral vision. Don't go nuts and create a mini-PRP all at once, however, because that may undo everything you are trying to accomplish by causing increased macular edema. (Lots more on the effect of a PRP on macular edema in Chapters 14 and 16.)

MOVING into the zone

The ETDRS recommended treating up to 500 microns from the center of the fovea, but this is close, and you may want to play it safe and stay 750 microns from the center in order to avoid trouble. This is an easy number to define—just mentally split the diameter of the disc in half, and put one end at the center of the fovea. Until you have a lot of experience, or become cavalier (usually they are the same), it is best to avoid getting close to the center. This is where observant patients can really get frustrated, because they can detect your spots more easily. It is also where you can do some serious damage to the perifoveal capillary network if you are not careful. A detailed angiogram is crucial before you work in this close, because you really need to be sure that you are not accidentally treating microaneurysms that happen to supply the few remaining capillaries that supply the fovea. If you shut them down, you can knock off large chunks of central vision, which is A Bad Thing.

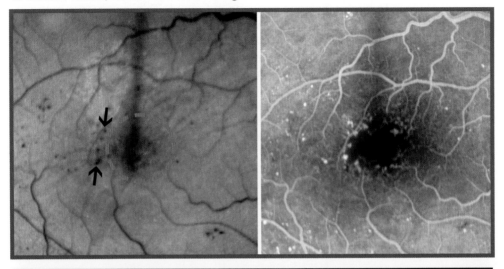

Figure 10. This is why it is good to have an FA before treating near the fovea. The circle represents an estimate of 500 microns from the fovea based on the patient's nerve. The microaneurysms temporal to the fovea (between the arrows) are far enough away to be treatable if you decide to follow ETDRS guidelines. However, you can see from the FA that aggressive treatment of these little devils could shut down the only vessels supplying the entire temporal side of the fovea—you could cause a lot of vision loss. (Extra credit if you notice that the brightest microaneurysm on the FA is not the same as the most obvious microaneurysm clinically.)

Although the ETDRS allowed treatment to within 300 microns of the fovea if necessary, if you really feel that you just *have* to treat closer than 700 microns, you may want to get a second opinion first. You will find an occasional patient that has a few big leakers near the foveal avascular zone, and gentle treatment directed only at the microaneurysms may fix the problem. In general, however, bad leaks in this area don't tend to respond to laser, especially if the fovea is cystic. You may need to consider intravitreal therapy, if it is available. (Such therapy was not available when the ETDRS was performed, and laser was the only way to try to dry up foveal edema—hence the more desperate treatment guidelines.) Definitely consider getting an OCT, too. Patients may have subtle traction that is keeping the fovea thick, and the vascular changes may be only bit players; ruling traction out first may save a lot of hassle. Remember that spots this close to the fovea will grow—are you sure that everyone will be happy with the results in five years if they spread into the fovea? Finally, never forget that any patient with refractory edema may actually have a bigger problem, such as accelerated hypertension or early renal failure. No perifoveal laser is going to replace nephrons—so think globally before acting locally on juxtafoveal RPE.

CODA...

The goal of life is to seek a balance between extremes. This is very true in the setting of laser treatment for diabetic macular edema. There is no question that very heavy treatment seems to be effective in eliminating edema (no retina = no edema), but can also create more problems with scotomas, decreased vision, and late complications. Lighter treatment decreases the risks of treatment, but also engenders the risk of permanent damage from incompletely treated macular edema. The best way to judge the needs of an individual patient's retina is experience, and if you end up treating a lot of diabetics you will develop a good sense for this. Until then, take heart—perhaps the most reasonable approach is to be very conservative in your treatments and follow the patients closely, retreating as necessary. There is probably more damage done by overly aggressive treatment of focal disease than by delayed treatment of focal disease. An upcoming chapter will try to give you some idea of what to watch for and when to bail out on patients with difficult-to-control macular disease. But first, a colorful box break followed by a mini-chapter on advanced laser techniques.

SOMETIMES AN ANGIOGRAM HAS A CHEATIN' HEART

Although the angiogram is usually your friend, there are times it can deceive you. For instance, patients may have "compensated" leakage on the FA. This means that they can have areas of leakage in the later phases, but that somehow the retina and RPE are able to pump the leakage out fast enough so that there is no secondary swelling of the retina. In other words, the angiogram may indicate there are areas that need to be treated but if you look closely at the retina with your own eyes there is actually no thickening and therefore no "clinically significant" macular edema.

Sometimes these areas of compensated leakage will have subtle thickening on OCT that is not apparent on clinical exam, or there may be early cystic changes on the OCT without any thickening. If these OCT findings are present it may justify treatment, but you must remember that the original ETDRS did not use OCT to determine who gets treated—only the clinical exam. Although treating patients based on a combination of FA and OCT findings alone—without clinically apparent thickening—seems reasonable it is not supported by a randomized trial yet. Proceed with caution.

Another way an angiogram can mess you up is with the diffuse leakage that can occur at the site of previous laser scars. These areas almost always stain into the later phases and you can really chase your tail if you keep hammering laser into these areas thinking that there is still leakage to treat (not to mention the fact that you will create large patches of atrophic retina and RPE). Again, look at the patient. Usually areas of previous laser treatment will be flatter and therefore do not need to be treated—even if they are leaking on the FA. If they are swollen in spite of previous treatment then you and the patient have a problem. If the previous laser is light then you can add some more. If there is a lot of laser you do not want to be beating the proverbial dead horse and blindly keep killing RPE—it may be time to think about other treatments such as intravitreal therapy or to re-evaluate the patient for subtle traction or a systemic problem that is causing trouble.

References and Suggested Reading

1.	Fong DS, Strauber SF, Aiello LP, et al. Comparison of the modified Early Treatment Diabetic Retinopathy Study and mild macular grid laser photocoagulation strategies for diabetic macular edema. Arch Ophthalmol. Apr 2007;125(4):469-480.

Folk JC, Pulido JS. Laser photocoagulation of the retina and choroid. San Francisco: American Academy of Ophthalmology, 1997.

Chew EY, Ferris FL III. Nonproliferative Diabetic Retinopathy. In: Ryan SJ. Retina, 4th ed. Philadelphia: Elsevier Mosby, 2006:v.2, pp 1271-1284.

Techniques for scatter and local photocoagulation treatment of diabetic retinopathy: Early Treatment Diabetic Retinopathy Study Report no. 3. The Early Treatment Diabetic Retinopathy Study Research Group. Int Ophthalmol Clin 1987;27:254-64.

Photocoagulation for diabetic macular edema: Early Treatment Diabetic Retinopathy Study Report no. 4. The Early Treatment Diabetic Retinopathy Study Research Group. Int Ophthalmol Clin 1987;27:265-72.

Case reports to accompany Early Treatment Diabetic Retinopathy Study Reports 3 and 4. The Early Treatment Diabetic Retinopathy Study Research Group. Int Ophthalmol Clin 1987;27:273-333.

Neubauer AS, Ulbig MW. Laser treatment in diabetic retinopathy. Ophthalmologica 2007;221:95-102.

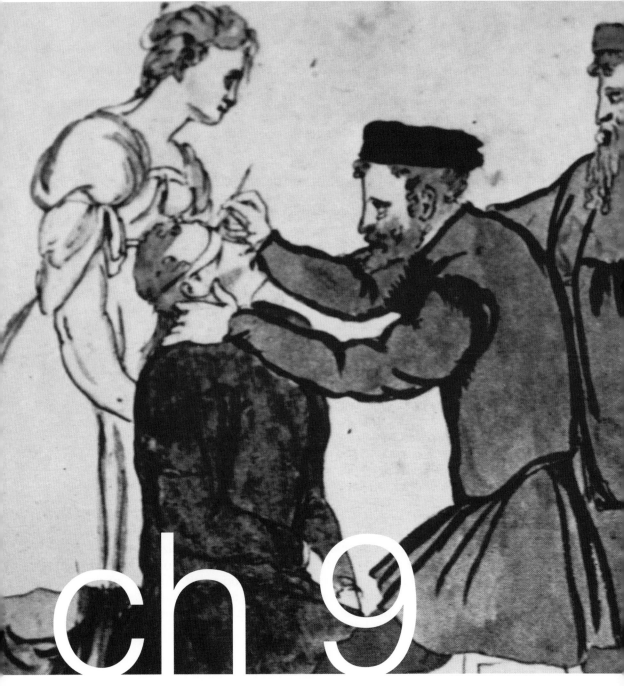

ch 9

Lasers 202

LASERS 202

It can get quite tedious if you need to constantly adjust your spot size and power in a patient with variably thickened retina and variable pigmentation. Reaching over to change the setting and then relocating yourself on the patient's retina can add a huge amount of time and frustration to the process for both yourself and the patient. There are some tricks you can use to avoid fussing with the laser settings for each spot—but they take a bit of experience. First of all, always strive to get the tightest, most consistent focus on your aiming beam. The energy delivery of your laser is totally dependent on this; if your spot is shifting and blurring, you are wasting your time—and you may even be dangerous if you are turning up the power for a blurry spot, and then suddenly the spot snaps into perfect focus. A consistently good aiming beam can seem impossible at first. Just practice—even if it means putting a contact lens on every patient (as well as family members, friends and each other). You don't even need to do it at the laser—practicing with the lenses in the clinic will readily pay off when you switch to using them in the laser suite. The quicker this skill is internalized, the better it is for everyone. Just Do It.

Once you have mastered the art of seeing what you need to see, though, there are some tricks that can come in really handy for enhancing your laser skills. The first technique is to actually undo what you have learned. You have a great deal of control over the energy density when you defocus the spot in a controlled manner. This can be done by either moving the slit lamp back and forth or by throwing a little astigmatism into the lens by tilting it a bit (the former is more predictable and controllable). For instance, if you are doing a grid and moving into a thinner or more pigmented area, where you know your laser spot will be getting hotter, you can just defocus a bit and titrate the uptake without fiddling with the power knob. If you are working near the fovea you obviously do not want to be smearing out and enlarging your spot—it is much better to manually back off on the power—but everywhere else this can be a real time saver. Some older lasers are focused in a way that creates a cone of light, and by pushing the slit lamp in, you defocus. When you pull back, the spot size actually gets smaller, with a higher power density. This allows you a great deal of control, but you have to be careful if you tighten up the spot too much—for reasons that should not need mentioning by now. By the way, this technique is easier with an indirect contact lens. A direct lens does not focus and defocus the aiming beam as much, but you can still try it.

There is another variable that is even easier to work with, though, and that is the duration of the burn. If you work with a slightly longer time, say .15 or .2 seconds, you will be surprised at how easily you can control, with the pedal, the actual time the laser is on. In fact, if you get good at this, you will find that your foot can be much faster than even shorter durations, such as .1 second. You can then use your foot to titrate the burn—a quick hit for a light burn and more sustained pedal-to-metal for a longer, hotter burn if you run into thicker retina or paler RPE. (Remember, however, that if you are using longer durations you may run into trouble if the patient moves during a burn—but if you are light on your foot to begin with, you can usually react in time.)

It is not difficult to control both of these variables at the same time. You can continuously alter the spot focus and duration, and you can often do an entire laser without adjusting the settings.

Where can you quickly become experienced in this? Take a look at the PRP chapter. Over there, you can try out these techniques while you are doing several hundred spots and super-accuracy is not crucial. It doesn't take long to get a feel for these techniques under those circumstances, and it is a good way to avoid getting bored while doing a PRP.

If you can master these techniques, it will greatly improve your efficiency and safety—because you will have a much more intuitive feel for what the laser is doing and how you can control it. You will also be able to win friends, influence people, have great sex and make your wildest dreams come true. Can doctors who use lasers all day to correct refractive errors make that claim? Not likely…

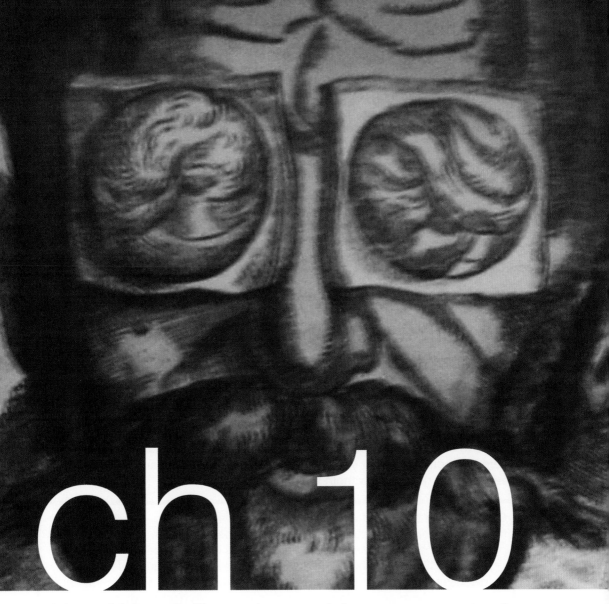

ch 10

Now What? Post-Laser Management of Macular Edema

NOW WHAT? Post-Laser Management of Macular Edema

Upon finishing the laser, take a moment to give the patient some post-op "instructions." Even though there really is nothing they need to do or not do after a macular laser, patients may fill this void with all kinds of self-imposed restrictions, depending often on what family and friends tell them. It is important to remind them that there are no activity restrictions subsequent to the laser. Patients are often worried that if they strain or lift they will burst the little blood vessels that you have just sealed. You want to reassure them that this is not the case at all. They have also been told for years that if they use their eyes too much, they will go blind or something. It is amazing how many patients will restrict their lives by trying to "rest their eyes," when it makes no difference whatsoever how they use them. Even if they don't ask you about it, you should always take the time to reassure patients that they cannot hurt their eyes by using them. The concept that one can damage one's eyes by straining them is so ingrained, especially in older patients, that you may find them asking about visual restrictions on a regular basis.

You should remind them that their eyes may be a bit scratchy. (Artificial tear samples come in handy here—patients may even feel that they actually received something of value if they walk out of the office with a free bottle in their hand.) Their eyes will often be blurry for a few days—sometimes a week or so—and they need to be warned about that as well. You should also remind them, once again, that you aren't doing Lasik and that the goal is to slow things down—they cannot expect to suddenly get better after the laser (reread Chapter 6, if necessary).

Most of the studies and texts suggest seeing the patients in three to four months. This is probably reasonable, because usually you will not begin to detect definite changes until this amount of time has passed. On the other hand, if someone just fiddled with your primary sense organ, would you really want to be told to come back in four months and good luck? Especially if you are being treated for something that you may not be symptomatic for, and that you have been told can get worse without you knowing it?

> **Cynically,** the three- to four-month time frame is also reasonable from a financial standpoint, because Medicare and most insurance companies won't pay squat for an office visit within three months of a laser treatment. (This is known as a "90-day global"—the surgical fee includes 90 days of follow-up.) As discussed in the next paragraph, it does make sense to see them sooner, but because there are no ironclad guidelines you can decide what you think is best for yourself and the individual patient. The point is that as you develop your own approach to follow-up, you want to be able to periodically look into your soul and feel comfortable that you are always serving the best interests of the patient and not just serving mammon. Whatever mammon is…

It may be reasonable to bring these patients back a little bit sooner, perhaps in six to eight weeks, simply to review the nature of the disease and the treatment and to make absolutely sure things are not deteriorating unexpectedly. This is especially important in patients who have one eye that is seeing much better than the eye you have treated—such patients may not know if their bad eye is getting worse, because the brain "covers" any blurriness with the vision from the good eye. The early visit also gives you a chance to head off any unhappiness patients may have with the success of the treatment by reminding them about the goals of treating macular edema. (If you are getting a sense that you have to repeat this every visit, you are right.) Finally, even if you can't detect much difference in the eye, you can at least tell the patient that things are stabilizing, which is always encouraging. By the way, don't forget to take the opportunity to nag the patient about their systemic control.

Of course, if the patient has worrisome disease, such as early cystic changes or hard exudates trying to build up in the fovea, you definitely want to bring them back sooner than three months. These are patients who need close follow-up, because if things are going downhill you will need to consider more aggressive measures such as intravitreal therapy. If patients have this type of problem, you don't want to wait to let chronic damage build up. (See the next chapter.)

Speaking about follow up, here is another useful tip: Get on the phone yourself and call the patient about a week after the treatment. Patients may have minor questions that they forgot to ask you, and you can address any issues they have. You will also be surprised about how many patients will say, "Gee, doc, things are not better yet," meaning, "I realize you told me not to expect any improvement and that the goal is to slow things down, but I still thought that I was supposed to be able to throw away my reading glasses after your laser." In response, you can once again review the philosophy of treating diabetic retinopathy. Finally, patients will be blown away that you took the time to check on them. When you do cataract surgery or Lasik, the patient can see for themselves the benefit of your efforts. Diabetic retinopathy patients do not usually get this type of reinforcement, and it is reassuring for them to know that you are concerned enough to make the extra effort to communicate.

Some of the toughest patients are those who return with some degree of persistent edema. The original ETDRS protocol called for repeat treatments until the edema had resolved. This ideal goal always sounded really good, but is sometimes far more difficult to achieve than textbooks would have you think. Traditionally, these patients were treated every three months until "the macula was dry." You will rapidly learn that for some patients this approach will vaporize the posterior pole. Often the decision to re-treat is more complex and becomes a balancing act between six factors:

1. The patient's perception of how they are doing (yes, you have to take a history, darn it).
2. The visual acuity.
3. The appearance of the retina relative to the pretreatment appearance.
4. Where the swelling is.
5. How much treatment has been placed.
6. Efforts the patient is taking to improve their control.

> **The next section** is talking about mild edema that is peripheral, without a lot of foveal changes. If you are dealing with bad foveal edema and crashing vision, you should not dilly-dally—you should either treat aggressively or refer the patient, depending on your situation.

If you feel the retina is not responding when you see the patient in follow-up, then the traditional approach is to keep treating them with laser—and a recent study suggests that, in general, this is still the gold standard.[1] However, recognize that if the patient feels they are doing well (and their vision is stable), it may be reasonable to monitor them a bit without treatment. You want to be sensitive to the fact that the patient may be getting fairly frustrated with the whole process—they are going through a lot of effort (and cost) with nothing to show for it as far as they can tell. If you just keep hammering away as a knee-jerk reflex, especially if the patient thinks they are stable, you may lose your most valuable asset: the patient's trust. You do not want them to get fed up with the process so much that they refuse to come back; they will end up with much worse disease when they finally return in a year or two with symptomatic vision loss.

As a result, careful observation can sometimes be the best approach, especially if they are getting their diabetes under better control. You may find that your treatment will work surprisingly well if you just give it more time than the textbooks say, and if your patient's hemoglobin A1c is sweet. (Perhaps "unsweet" would be a better adjective in this situation—more on this issue in Chapter 20.)

If you watch such patients closely and re-treat parsimoniously, then the patient is much more likely to understand what you are doing, and is therefore more likely to stick with you for the long term. Your treatment will also be much less destructive than if you had continued to treat at every visit simply because there was some persistent swelling. Obviously, you don't want to wait months if you think the retina is not as good as it should be—you want to bring these patients back soon, so that if they don't improve you can jump in and do the treatment as often as necessary.

This is where some sort of visual aid, such as a convincing OCT or photos of hard exudates driving towards the macula, can be very helpful. If you have to repeatedly treat a patient who has no symptoms, you can help them to understand the importance of close follow-up by showing them what you are treating. Hopefully they will understand that what they perceive with their vision does not reflect the reality of the situation.

> **If you think** the patient is just not getting it when it comes to additional treatment, it is a good time to consider a second opinion. Even if you don't need one, it is always a good idea to assuage any concerns that the patient might have before they go out and do it on their own.

Please understand that this discussion does not advocate blowing off a retina that is not improving after treatment. There are some patients that simply need recurrent aggressive treatment to bring things under control. The point is that you need to be flexible with your approach, and keep in mind all of the six factors mentioned above when assessing the patient. Some patients, especially less sophisticated ones, are not as with you as you may think, and you should be prepared to treat the patient's head and not just their retina in order to keep from losing them altogether. As long as you watch the retinal morphology carefully, you can bend the rules and monitor patients without continually treating them just because the ETDRS toldja to.

What kind of testing do you need to do on follow up? Although some experts will get an OCT and perhaps even an angiogram at each visit, it is hard to justify all that testing unless things are going downhill. It turns out that numbers one through six above come down to simply talking to and examining the patient, which is often all that is necessary. If you are not sure how the patient is doing, an OCT can be an invaluable and risk-free way to find out and you can use the results to show the patient exactly how bad things are.

An angiogram is usually not necessary unless the eye is worsening and one needs to know whether there are a lot of new leaks and where they are (i.e., a bunch of leaks at the edge of the foveal avascular zone mean it is time for intravitreal treatment; a bunch of new leaks to the side allows precise focal treatment without unnecessary retinal destruction). Of course, if you do not have access to such testing then you have to rely on your clinical skills—which can be almost as good as the most expensive imaging equipment if you are a careful observer.

Some screwball things to watch for:

1. Blowing out the macula with too much treatment all at once. This was covered in Chapter 8, but it is worth repeating. Sometimes you can get carried away on a patient with lots of little microaneurysms and put in a ton of treatment because it is, well, fun, and you really feel like you are helping. These patients can come back a lot worse—you can literally push the edema right into the fovea. Usually you do not see these patients at the routine follow up visit. They tend to come in, quite unhappily, a week or two after your treatment. Just remember to go easy and don't end up in this fix.

2. A paradoxical increase in hard exudates. There are occasional patients who demonstrate a very annoying tendency to increase their hard exudates subsequent to treatment—even though the retina is actually better. This probably represents transient accumulation of hard exudates as the interstitial fluid is pumped out and protein and fats are left behind. However, it is really annoying to put in a beautiful treatment and, two months later, have 50% more hard exudates all over the place. The key here is to look at the retinal thickness and the vision, both of which should be stable to improved. If there is increased retinal thickening, then the hard exudates are worse because the patient is worse, and your treatment is not holding it back. If the retina otherwise looks good and you think you are dealing with this particular situation, it is reasonable to obtain photographs and check the patient in about six weeks.

3. Sometimes patients can have transient worsening of their macular

edema subsequent to a severe systemic illness, such as a hospital admission for cardiac problems or for a significant infection. These patients may spontaneously improve over a couple of months as they recover, and it is reasonable to watch such patients a bit before automatically treating them (assuming they do not have a really worrisome morphology such as hard exudates streaming into the fovea or marked vision loss).

What if things are clearly going downhill?

If this is happening, you first need to make sure the patient's systemic risk factors are under control. If you are not getting the information you need from the patient or the patient's doctor, you should do your own evaluation. This would include checking the labs, such as hemoglobin A1c, lipids, CBC and renal studies, and checking the blood pressure yourself. Do not *ever* underestimate the importance of systemic control. It is amazing how a hopeless-looking macula can turn around with a combination of laser treatment and aggressive systemic management. Conversely, it can be very frustrating to treat patients who are cavalier about their control and listen to them complain that your lasers aren't helping them as they spring leak after leak in their macula.

Also, don't forget to check whether they are on one of the glitazone family of oral hypoglycemic agents. These can cause fluid retention and heart failure, and are thought to cause worsening of macular edema.[2] Patients whose macular edema is exacerbated by these medications usually have problems with systemic edema, but it can rarely happen without obvious fluid retention so you should consider this in any patient who has refractory cystic macular edema. You have to be careful—you don't want to scare the patient so much they stop taking the med on their own. You also don't want to demand that the medical physician stop these drugs on everyone whom you are treating for macular edema. You can cause a lot of trouble if doctors try to switch these patients to something else, and there is no data to suggest that there is some sort of universal effect on all diabetics. If anything, this side effect is relatively rare. The point is to at least think about this if you are having trouble controlling a patient's retinal swelling. Go to blue box land for a list of the glitazones…

The Glitazones (or, more unpronounceably, The Thiazolidinediones):

As monotherapy:
Rosiglitazone (Avandia)
Pioglitazone (Actos)

As combination pills:
Rosiglitazone and metformin (Avandamet)
Rosiglitazone and glimepiride (Avandaryl)
Pioglitazone and metformin (Actoplus Met)

The handy thing to remember is that these are about the only oral hypoglycemics that start with the letter "A." (OK, for completeness, the other A-pills are: acetohexamide (Dymelor) and glimepride (Amaryl). Neither of these is associated with macular edema—acetohexamide is no longer available in the USA and glimepride is not a glitazone.)

There are some other things you must consider in patients who are not responding well to laser treatment. A common problem—once again—is some sort of traction that is pulling up on the retina and keeping it swollen. This can be due to an obvious epiretinal membrane or a more subtle process related to vitreous contraction. The diabetic vitreous tends to be exceptionally sticky, and it can remain attached to the macula as it tries to contract due to normal aging and structural changes caused by the retinopathy. As it tightens it pulls on the macula, creating edema that tends to be very diffuse, cystic, and refractory to laser. Sometimes you can suspect this on clinical examination because there is a golden sheen overlying the retina that is best seen with a contact lens. These patients also tend to have far more leakage on the angiogram than one would suspect from the amount of retinopathy present. There may even be macular distortion if there is an associated epiretinal membrane or incomplete vitreous detachment. However, many times, subtle traction will not be visible on clinical examination, and OCT testing can be invaluable because the vitreous inserting on the retina will be very obvious. (Figure 1 in Chapter 18 is an example.) In fact, if you don't have access to an OCT, you should send the patient out for one, because it is much better to find subtle traction rather than keep repeating lasers that will not work well at all. The presence of traction mandates referral to a retinal specialist, because patients presenting with it may benefit from vitrectomy. (Chapter 18 discusses this and other reasons for referral for vitrectomy.)

Also, it is worth reviewing Chapter 26 on differential diagnosis when faced with refractory macular edema. There are other things to consider, both systemic and intraocular, that can mimic or worsen retinopathy and if you miss them you will be wasting your time doing fruitless lasers.

Finally, there are some patients who just keep springing leaks and just keep needing more treatment. It can be very rewarding to gently treat each new area and keep someone seeing for years and years. Your job as a comprehensive ophthalmologist is to be sure that you are not just eliminating perifoveal retina with lots of enthusiastic laser when the patient might benefit from treatment with another modality—whether it be better systemic control, vitrectomy or intravitreal therapy. (The latter happens to be the subject of the next chapter—and this would have been a nice segue except for the following sections.)

CHAPTER 10.1 Additional Bits That Don't Quite Fit Anywhere Else

Doc, my vision is really blurry in the morning...

If patients develop edema that is in or around the fovea, you will often hear the above complaint. There are a few things you should consider when patients tell you this.

First of all, OCT studies have suggested that macular edema is worse in the morning, presumably because the retina swells during the night, just like someone's ankles swell up if they spend a lot of time standing.[3] Does this mean that they should sleep with a few pillows? No one has looked at this. Maybe you could do an ARVO project…

Another reason may be that their glucose is getting low in the early morning, and by the time they wake up, it has rebounded a bit (kind of a mini-Somogyi phenomenon*). You will find that many diabetics, once they have significant retinopathy, will tell you that their vision gets blurry when their glucose gets a bit on the low side—not bad enough to give them the shakes or sweats, but their "weakened" retina seems to become especially sensitive to an otherwise unnoticeable drop in glucose. Indeed, for many patients this becomes a new way to tell that they need to check their sugar. The point is that you may want to suggest that patients set their alarm a few hours earlier than normal to do a fingerstick glucose. If the glucose is on the low side it may be contributing to their morning blur, and they may want to review their management with their medical doctor to see whether they can minimize their symptoms.

*Remember, this is the thing where diabetics get low glucose during the night, and then compensatory mechanisms kick in and jack up the sugar by the time they awaken and check their glucose. Because the AM glucose is high, the doctor increases the PM insulin, which only makes the problem worse, and a vicious cycle ensues.

Don't forget non-retinal things, too. Sometimes patients will have a bit of dry eye that makes the tear film rusty in the morning—especially if they have superimposed lid problems like a lagophthalmos or floppy eyelid syndrome (the latter is not uncommon in obese elderly diabetics). Another possibility could be early Fuchs corneal dystrophy. Your friendly neighborhood retina specialist will usually not think of this kind of stuff, so please protect your patient from our ignorance by being a good generalist and considering it.

There may be another reason that has no scientific basis whatsoever, but it sounds really good simply because there are sooo many patients, with all types of macular disease, who tell you their vision is blurry in the morning. There seems to be a part of the brain in charge of "Photoshopping" the world, and that part expects to have crisp vision upon awakening—as it has for the bulk of a patient's life. When it is suddenly faced with the kind of crummy vision that damaged maculae provide, it takes it a while do some image processing to overcome the ragged input it is getting—almost like overcoming morning stiffness by getting up and moving around. OK, this explanation looks really lame in print, but it plays well with patients—especially if you have ruled out any pathology. Go write your own book if you don't like it…

CHAPTER 10.2

Refractory Diabetic Macular Edema in Places with No Specialists
(Remember, this book is not just for decadent docs in developed countries.)

What if you only have the option of doing laser—no intravitreal treatment or vitrectomy? One might hope a race of thoughtful aliens will take over our planet and equalize the distribution of healthcare, so that no human being is treated worse than another. Until then, however, here are some suggestions.

First of all, if you really are the only one around, then it would be great if you could get some extra training, because your local population would benefit. Can you spend a week at a specialty center and learn some tricks and tips? Can you get a local service club (like the Lions or Rotarians) to help with cost? Some of the resources mentioned in Chapter 6 can help with additional education and training.

Second, it is likely that you are also in a situation where the medical control of your patients is dismal. As mentioned numerous times in this book, anything you do will not work as well if the patients are not well controlled. If there is anything that can be done to help with this, it will make your life a lot easier.

Third, if you are in this situation it is likely that patients are showing up late in their disease course, which only makes your job more impossible. Try to do anything to get them in sooner—patient and doctor education, assistance from service and religious organizations, telemedicine screening—whatever.

As for treating the patient with laser alone, there are not a lot of options beyond adding more spots as patients get worse. You need to do this parsimoniously, though. It has been suggested that once you put about 300 to 400 small spots into a posterior pole, you have done about as much as you can hope for with laser. Numbers like this came from the bad old days—before there were other treatments. Try not to go this high if possible, because this many spots will definitely expand and start to cause problems if the patient lives for many years (although you may not need to worry about this as much in developing countries, where diabetics tend to die sooner). If you are using very small light spots, though, it may be possible to perform multiple treatments, especially if you are just doing focal treatment directed at new microaneurysms.

Sadly, if you really are in this boat you are probably just barely staying ahead of your patient load, and you are also likely seeing lots of really bad, puffed-up maculas. In this situation, you are simply trying to keep eyes in the 20/400 range and not let patients go all the way to hand motions from macular disease. You also need conserve your resources—if you do gentle, staged treatment on everyone, you can get so backlogged with following them that you can't take care of anyone else. This situation may be the one time when your best option is to do a grid of 100 to 150 spots and hope for the best, and then repeat as needed until you have put in about 300 to 400 spots total. Again, this is not ideal at all, but if there are no other solutions, this approach at least gets enough scarring in to help keep the retina from totally swelling up. Patient expectations are also crucial if you are forced to do this. They must understand that they will get worse no matter what you do—it is just that by treating them, you will hopefully hold on to as much vision as possible. (The last part of Chapter 6 reviews this in more detail.)

It may be tempting to treat patients with intravitreal steroids in this situation, but you need to give serious thought to the potential complications. What are your options if a patient gets into trouble? If there is no way to treat it, a case of endophthalmitis or retinal detachment or refractory glaucoma is far worse than count-fingers vision from macular edema. This is not to say that one should never try intravitreal therapy but rather that you need to carefully balance all the risks if you have limited resources.

> **Unfortunately**, there are some doctors in developed countries who do have access to specialists but act like they don't—until a patient's retina is far gone. The approach for such folks seems to be: "How can I extract the maximum amount of money from a patient before I refer them out and don't get a chance to bill them again?" One hopes that they are not really thinking this, and that they are simply deluding themselves into thinking they know what is best for the patient without paying attention to the literature (not that thinking this is much of an improvement over greed). If you know someone like this, we can send them a free copy of this book (with anonymous return address) if you wish. Here is the point: Do the best you can but if you think you are getting in over your head don't hesitate to ask for help. You—and your patient—will sleep better.

References and Suggested Reading

1.   Diabetic Retinopathy Clinical Research Network. A Randomized Trial Comparing Intravitreal Triamcinolone Acetonide and Focal/Grid Photocoagulation for Diabetic Macular Edema. Ophthalmology. 2008 Sep;115(9):1447-9.

2.   Ryan EH, Jr., Han DP, Ramsay RC, et al. Diabetic macular edema associated with glitazone use. Retina 2006;26:562-70.

3.   Polito A, Del Borrello M, Polini G, Furlan F, Isola M, Bandello F. Diurnal variation in clinically significant diabetic macular edema measured by the Stratus OCT. Retina 2006;26:14-20.

Folk JC, Pulido JS. Laser photocoagulation of the retina and choroid. San Francisco: American Academy of Ophthalmology, 1997.

Treatment techniques and clinical guidelines for photocoagulation of diabetic macular edema. Early Treatment Diabetic Retinopathy Study Report Number 2. Early Treatment Diabetic Retinopathy Study Research Group. Ophthalmology 1987;94:761-74.

ch 11

Intravitreal Therapy and How It
Fits Into Your Armamentarium.
Or Not.

Although laser has historically been the mainstay of treatment of diabetic retinopathy, there is now tremendous interest in the use of intravitreal therapy to help control the damage. As of this writing, there is no single proven approach for using intravitreal drugs, so it is hard to provide firm guidelines. Furthermore, intravitreal treatment can significantly change the risk-benefit ratio given the potential complications, especially if you are practicing in an area where there may be limited resources to address such complications. For instance, if you are at an academic center where you can walk your patient with steroid-induced glaucoma down the hall to a world expert on glaucoma, your risk-benefit ratio may be very different than if you are practicing in a smaller town where the same patient may be operated on by someone who does only 10 filters a year. Finally, it is likely that some readers will not have access to specialty care at all.

As a result, this chapter will simply give an overview of these drugs with some suggestions about how they might fit in to the treatment of diabetic retinopathy. A complete discussion of the rationale, pharmacology, techniques and risks is beyond the scope of this book, but if you are going to use intravitreal therapy, you *have* to become more familiar with all of these issues—do not stop with the information here. Ultimately, you will need to decide whether you want to use these medications; this will be determined by their availability, your level of comfort, and your ability to identify and deal with complications. The philosophy of your local retinal community is also very important, and you will need to figure this out on your own—especially in terms of when to refer if you do not use these techniques. Hopefully, there will be studies over the next few years that will give us all a definite idea of the best way to use these drugs, in the same way the Diabetic Retinopathy Study and the Early Treatment of Diabetic Retinopathy Study have helped to define the use of lasers.

INTRAVITREAL THERAPY & MACULAR EDEMA Triamcinolone and Avastin

Triamcinolone Acetonide

Steroids seem to be the ultimate "Radiator Stop Leak" for perifoveal capillaries. People initially went berserk when it became apparent that this drug could have a dramatic effect on reversing central cystic diabetic macular edema—something for which laser alone is often frustratingly ineffective. However, with time, it has become apparent that for many patients the initial positive response seems to gradually weaken, and the long-term results are less stunning. A recent study even suggested that laser is still better than triamcinolone alone for many patients.[1] When you add in the inevitable cataract and risk of glaucoma, one begins to realize that this is not the miracle drug everyone at first thought it to be.

On the other hand, if used judiciously, it can be very effective in controlling central edema in selected patients.[2] Unfortunately, there is no good way to figure out which patients will benefit the most, and there are no long-term controlled trials that provide specific guidelines. There is, therefore, absolutely no consensus about how this drug fits into the management of macular edema. If you are in a situation where triamcinolone is unavailable, then you have to work with lasers. If it is available, then you really need to talk to your local specialists about how they feel it fits in. You don't want to turn into some sort of renegade outlier from either overuse or underuse. The trick is to decide which patients seem to do best with the drug, and then hope that the risk of cataract and glaucoma does not offset any apparent gains.

It is agreed that mild macular edema, especially if it is away from the fovea, should simply be treated with laser. Once the edema starts to build up in the fovea, there is a sense that, somewhere, a clock begins to start ticking; it seems that leaving a lot of edema in the fovea for an extended period of time decreases the ultimate visual recovery. How much time is too much time? No one knows. Perhaps a reasonable guess is three to six months, but that is total speculation, so if you find someone who feels differently, please feel free to scratch out the above numbers and write in your own.

The point is that if you try a laser or two and there is persistent edema in the fovea, then you do not want to keep lasering and waiting and lasering and waiting. It is best to get the patient to someone who can do intravitreal therapy before there is more and more permanent microarchitectural damage. You also need to factor in the rate of change in terms of how fast you refer. If the fovea is mildly thickened and the vision is OK, then time is on your side. If the fovea is a bubbly mess with hard exudates streaming in like Leeroy Jenkins, then you should send the patient sooner (Figure 1). There is definitely a sense that the magic drugs work better on fresh edema than on old chronic disease.

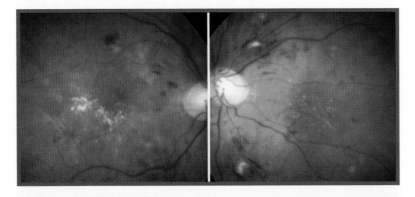

Figure 1. This patient presented with central cystic macular edema and a vision of 20/400 in the right eye and 20/80 in the left eye. The worrisome thing about this case is that the hard exudates are just starting to build up into the fovea. You can see that the right fovea will soon be swamped, and the left fovea has a very scary "sugar dusting" of exudates that means that it will soon follow. This pattern does not tend to do well with laser alone, so it is not a good idea to put in some laser and wait three to four months to see what happens — permanent damage can occur. This is the kind of patient who will likely need intravitreal therapy, if available.

Here is an example of one approach: If there is fairly significant foveal thickening (say, greater than 300 microns on OCT testing), and if the vision is starting to deteriorate (say 20/30 to 20/40), you might consider intravitreal therapy in order to jumpstart the eye and get the edema reversed as you are adding the laser. (There is a sense that the laser creates long-term control once the intravitreal treatment has produced transient improvement.) Note, however, that these acuities are definitely not absolute. For instance, older, retired patients may not want to take the risk of intravitreal treatment until they are 20/80, whereas younger, wired types may want a full-court press to stay 20/20. If the patient does want an injection, some doctors feel it may be better to inject first and then do the laser a week or two later. This is because once the retina is thinner, it is easier to treat without getting the large burns caused by scattering of the laser beam through thickened retina. If you adopt this approach, you also want to be sure you remember where the pathology is. Once you flatten the retina with a drug, it can be hard to tell where you needed to treat.

The one thing you must never do is to give a patient an injection just because you can. Please do not be seduced by the intense immediate gratification that occurs when you bring your first patient back for a pressure check and the edema is *gone* (and the patient is actually happy and smiling at you like, well, a Lasik patient). This experience creates powerful positive reinforcement that is not really justified. The long-term reality of intravitreal therapy is never as good as your "first time." Try to remember that by using this medication you are embarking on a process that may end up being very frustrating for you and the patient as the edema keeps coming back and the vision slowly slips away (and the cataract gets worse, and then you have to do cataract surgery on an eye with a weepy macula and elevated pressure). Also, remember that the pressure can rise insidiously, and this may show up well after the drug should have worn off.[3] If there is a concern about the pressure, it is reasonable to check the IOP periodically for perhaps a year or two after an injection. As a comprehensive ophthalmologist, this is particularly important to remember because your retina specialist may forget about this.

> By the way, although this chapter emphasizes the side effects that are particular to each drug, don't forget that the patient also has to accept the risks of the intravitreal injection itself. These risks include infection, sterile uveitis, vitreous hemorrhage, retinal detachment, and some really embarrassing things like intralenticular injection, suprachoroidal injection and wound rupture (i.e., if the patient had recent cataract surgery, corneal transplant or a thin filtering bleb). Although these complications are unlikely, the risk can add up since most patients need multiple treatments. As a wise retinal specialist once put it: "These aren't flu shots we're giving here."

In many ways, the use of intravitreal triamcinolone involves a search for those patients who seem to gain long-term benefit from the treatment. If you or your retina specialist tries the drug and the fovea dries up, but the vision doesn't improve, then such a patient is not an ideal candidate for continued therapy (especially if the pressure goes up). If the vision improves and the effect seems to be long-lasting, then such a patient may benefit greatly from intermittent injections combined with appropriate laser. If the results are somewhere in between—as is usually the case—then it comes down to the patient's wishes versus your sense of the long-term risk of chronic intravitreal steroid treatment.

Bevacizumab (Avastin) (and its expensive cousins)

The anti-vascular endothelial growth factor (anti-VEGF) drugs are also useful for treating macular edema. A real textbook could tell you why. Suffice it to say that blocking VEGF seems to seal leaky blood vessels. Studies involving the other anti-VEGF drugs—pegaptanib (Macugen) and ranibizumab (Lucentis)—have been performed or are under way. However, it is hard to imagine how any health-care system can survive if it has to pay for these drugs, especially for a chronic disease like diabetic retinopathy. For instance, at present there are a number of promising studies evaluating the effectiveness of Lucentis in diabetic macular edema. It is probable that results attributed to Lucentis will—right or wrong—end up being extrapolated to Avastin out of economic necessity, particularly in the developing world. Until there is definitive data indicating the two drugs are vastly different in effect, it is likely that Avastin will be the mainstay for treating diabetic retinopathy; it is certainly the cheapest and most commonly used drug in this category for now.

Although Avastin does appear to be effective in terms of reversing diabetic macular edema, there is a general sense that it is not as potent as triamcinolone. If triamcinolone is 10 on a scale of one to 10, then bevacizumab seems to come in between three and six. However, there is essentially no risk of glaucoma or cataract formation with Avastin, and surgeries to correct these latter two problems are not without risk in patients who have active retinopathy. On the other hand, there is concern with the anti-VEGF agents about systemic toxicity, such as thrombosis or stroke; right now, it is not clear at all whether this is a real concern, but it still needs to be discussed with the patient.

At this point, many texts will add something about how you should consult the patient's internist before administering anti-VEGF agents, especially because these patients are likely to have potential comorbidities such as heart disease or history of stroke. This seems like a reasonable thing to do—until you realize that there is no internist in the world who can predict the real risk of intravitreal anti-VEGF agents for any patient. It would even be impressive if the average internist had even heard of the use of anti-VEGF agents for retinopathy.

This is one of those weenie things that we do as ophthalmologists in order to avoid any real responsibility. Basically, your level of "freaked-out-ness" over covering yourself will help you decide how far you want to pursue this—but you are ultimately the one doing the injection, and it is your job to stay on top of the data and the patient's systemic status in order to make the best decision you can. (Besides, getting some sort of vague clearance to do an injection is really only pretend protection. Plaintiff attorneys love it when doctors start blaming each other.)

As with triamcinolone, there are no absolute guidelines about how Avastin fits into the treatment algorithm. Because Avastin has fewer ocular side effects, many folks will start treatment with Avastin and then move on to triamcinolone as needed, although one must be prepared to do more frequent injections when using Avastin alone. There are also multiple variations on any particular theme. For instance, some people will combine lower doses of Avastin and triamcinolone at the same time to try to maximize the benefit and minimize the side effects. This may be done with or without supplementary laser treatment—there are some papers that suggest such an approach is useful, and other papers that suggest it is not. Another approach is to try serial Avastin injections about a month apart, in hopes that sustained treatment will be more effective. Whatever you do, it makes sense to use the laser to treat obvious focal leaks and to do a light grid to diffuse leaks, because the laser can make permanent changes, whereas the intravitreal medications tend to be transient. But definitely go lightly with the photons. The whole point of the intravitreal drugs is to "train" the capillaries to stop leaking so that you do not have to treat as heavily with laser as you might if you didn't have this option. And no matter what drug you use or don't use in the vitreous, never forget the stuff in the upcoming paragraph:

Remember that nothing you do will work particularly well if you do not get the patient to pay close attention to their systemic vascular risk factors. Although you can go to Chapter 20 for the full scoop, with experience you will see how patients can "cure" central cystic macular edema with a combination of local ophthalmic treatment and improved systemic control. This may take a year or two, but it is exciting to watch patients begin to care for themselves and then watch their macular edema become less and less of a problem. You can give the sweetest intravitreal injections and do the finest macular laser, but if you don't emphasize systemic control with both patients and their physicians you are functioning at the Epsilon-Minus Semi-Moron level of doctorness.

Intravitreal Therapy and Proliferative Disease

Although there were some attempts to use triamcinolone to supplement the treatment of proliferative disease, it really does not have enough anti-neovascular power to be effective in this situation. Avastin, on the other hand, can be dramatically effective. Remember, however, that this drug simply changes the intraocular milieu on a temporary basis. You still need to do something to permanently change the inside of the eye in order to keep the bad chemicals away. If one uses Avastin to treat proliferative disease, the new vessels will simply return within a month or two as the Avastin wears off. As a result, you need to perform a plain-vanilla panretinal photocoagulation to get long-term control of the situation. Some argue that it is better to get total control with Avastin at first, because it will help protect the macula and allow you to work the PRP in gently—and it may allow faster disease control with less laser. No one knows yet whether this is really a better way; studies are being done to address the issue.

However, be *very* careful about injecting Avastin if there are large amounts of new vessels. It turns out that using Avastin to control proliferative disease can actually be very dangerous in the setting of extensive neovascularization. The drug will cause the vessels to contract forcefully and can result in very severe traction retinal detachments, which can be difficult or even impossible to fix. These can occur quite quickly, often within days or weeks of the injection. What should you consider "a lot" of neovascularization? Sorry, it is hard to be specific. One should probably start getting nervous about using Avastin if there is anything more than scattered little bushes of new vessels. Certainly, if there are large vessels up into the vitreous or broad sheets of vessels along the arcades or periphery, it gets very risky to use the stuff.

In such settings most doctors will get in a good PRP, and if the laser cannot completely control the process, then Avastin is used prior to vitrectomy to shrink up the blood vessels as much as possible and minimize intraoperative hemorrhaging. The Avastin injection is usually given less than a week before surgery, and the patient must understand that once the Avastin is given they have to go through with the surgery—you don't want to give it then have the surgery be cancelled due to medical instability.

> **There is, however,** one aspect of proliferative disease that pretty much everyone agrees is the perfect use for Avastin: if the patient has anterior segment neovascularization with neovascular glaucoma. Skip to Chapter 19 for more info...

Ultimately, the whole issue of intravitreal therapy in the setting of diabetic retinopathy is a brave new world with few definite guidelines. You get to decide whether you want to use these drugs or refer out—and you can also decide exactly what role you want them to play in your management. You have to pay close attention to the latest studies to be sure that you are not either over- or under-treating (or over- or under-referring) your patients. You also need to be the one to protect your patient from glaucoma as a result of triamcinolone because retina specialists can be really bad about this. Finally, never forget that even though these drugs can refreshingly dry up a macula in the short term, there is no treatment as good as making sure that patients take good care of themselves.

TO INFINITY & BEYOND Diabetic Retinopathy in the Future

This is a good time to point out that there are a lot of other drugs in the pipe-line—both for the eye and systemically—that may play a role in treating this disease. For instance, there are several sustained-release steroid implants being evaluated for use in diabetic retinopathy. It is likely that devices that slowly re-lease other drugs, such as the anti-VEGF agents, will soon be developed.

There are also modified laser techniques that may result in significant changes in how diabetics are treated. Micropulse laser was mentioned in Chapter 3, but there is also a suggestion that standard laser can be used to indirectly control macular edema. Because VEGF comes from the ischemic peripheral retina, and because VEGF causes vascular leakage, it is thought that by doing mild panreti-nal photocoagulation in peripheral ischemic retina, one can help control leakage in the macula. As we shall see in subsequent chapters, one is always worried that panretinal treatment will exacerbate macular edema, so this thinking seems a bit counterintuitive. In fact, such an approach is not even new—it was sug-gested years ago, but now it can be viewed in the context of what we know about VEGF activity.[4] This is not to say that everyone with macular edema needs a PRP—there are no studies yet that prove such an approach is valid. Rather, it is a reminder to keep an open mind and recognize that what we know "for sure" can easily change with time.

In terms of systemic therapy, the most obvious treatment is to simply address the patient's glucose control, as well as the other vascular risk factors discussed in Chapter 20. However, there are a host of other pathways that mediate the damage caused by diabetes, and a lot of research is directed toward finding drugs that can interfere with these pathways. For instance, protein kinase C subtype beta (PKC-beta) is an enzyme that is felt to contribute to diabetic micro-vascular damage when it is upregulated in hyperglycemic states. Ruboxistaurin is a PKC-beta inhibitor that was shown to have a mild effect on retinopathy. Un-fortunately, the results have not been good enough to justify FDA approval, and further studies are under way. It does serve, however, as exciting proof that it is possible to prevent damage by means other than laser and drugs in the eye.

Note of Caution: Diabetes is the leading cause of blindness in patients under the age of 65, and any treatment shown to be effective—even a little—stands to make someone an awful lot of coin. It is hoped that everyone is driven largely by a desire to make the world a better place, but one person's major breakthrough may be another person's marginal improvement—and sometimes throwing a lot of money into the mix does not help to get the reality pinned down.

You may have noticed this if you were reading the eye literature a few years ago, when preliminary trials were being done on ruboxistaurin. There were drug company advertisements that simply talked about the PKC-beta enzyme alone, seemingly as a way to prepare everyone's mind for the drug's release. There were also announce-ments of its effectiveness in the ophthalmic community—yet the FDA did not approve it and requested further studies.

The point is that although it is hard enough to be the best clinician one can be, more and more one has to also be able to look critically at the data as new treatments come online. It gets even tougher when one has to balance the benefits of new treat-ments against the cost to society at large—and now this box is getting way off topic. Back to work.

Other pathways under examination include those involving growth hormone, insulin-like growth factor, metalloproteases, and various mediators of inflammation. There is also work being done with advanced glycation endproducts (AGEs). These are produced in higher than normal levels during episodes of hyperglycemia, and they seem to play a role in diabetic microvascular damage. There is even a receptor for these compounds (the very appropriate acronym for this receptor is "RAGE") and activation of this receptor appears to elicit oxidative stress and inflammation in various cells. Interfering with all of these mechanisms will likely give us better and better ways to prevent diabetic damage of all types.

It is inevitable that in the future we may have a totally different philosophy when it comes to treating diabetic reinopathy. We may be using very light lasers—or perhaps no lasers at all—in conjunction with local and/or systemic drugs. You should keep your eye on the literature and stay abreast of new developments— these are exciting times, and our present treatments will, hopefully, be relegated to museum displays that sit next to exhibits on bleeding and purging. However, there are still a lot of patients who can benefit from old-school treatments, so on to the next manifestation of diabetic retinopathy: proliferative disease.

References and Suggested Reading

1.   Diabetic Retinopathy Clinical Research Network. A Randomized Trial Comparing Intravitreal Triamcinolone Acetonide and Focal/Grid Photocoagulation for Diabetic Macular Edema. Ophthalmology. 2008 Sep;115(9):1447-9.

2.   Gillies MC, Sutter FK, Simpson JM, Larsson J, Ali H, Zhu M. Intravitreal triamcinolone for refractory diabetic macular edema: two-year results of a double-masked, placebo-controlled, randomized clinical trial. Ophthalmology 2006;113:1533-8.

3.   Williams CP, Konstantopoulos A, Rowley SA, Luff AJ. Late intraocular pressure rise following intravitreal triamcinolone injection. Clin Experiment Ophthalmol 2007;35:385-6.

4.   Gardner TW, Eller AW, Friberg TR. Reduction of severe macular edema in eyes with poor vision after panretinal photocoagulation for proliferative diabetic retinopathy. Graefes Arch Clin Exp Ophthalmol 1991;229:323-8.

Cunningham MA, Edelman JL, Kaushal S. Intravitreal steroids for macular edema: the past, the present, and the future. Surv Ophthalmol 2008;53:139-49.

Grover D, Li TJ, Chong CC. Intravitreal steroids for macular edema in diabetes. Cochrane Database Syst Rev 2008:CD005656.

Furlani BA, Meyer CH, Rodrigues EB, et al. Emerging pharmacotherapies for diabetic macular edema. Expert Opin Emerg Drugs 2007;12:591-603.

Mohamed Q, Gillies MC, Wong TY. Management of diabetic retinopathy: a systematic review. JAMA 2007;298:902-16.

Tremolada G, Lattanzio R, Mazzolari G, Zerbini G. The therapeutic potential of VEGF inhibition in diabetic microvascular complications. Am J Cardiovasc Drugs 2007;7:393-8.

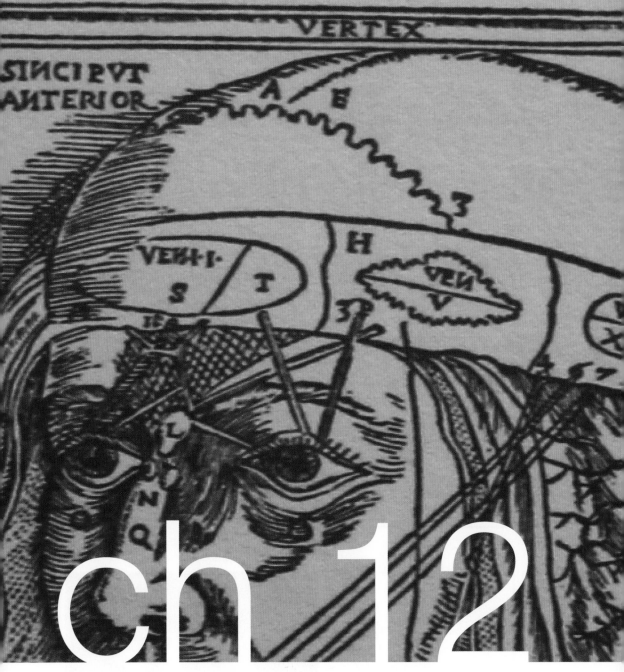

ch 12

Proliferative Diabetic Retinopathy and Other Things That Go Bump in the Night

THE NUMBERS

Proliferative diabetic retinopathy (PDR) is the real bad boy—it can make an eye stone-black blind. It tends to occur more often and more severely in younger patients with Type 1 diabetes, although no diabetic demographic is free from this problem. In general, the presence of proliferative disease is correlated to the duration of diabetes. For Type 1 patients, the risk is up to 50% if they have had diabetes for 20 years or more. Proliferative disease tends to be less frequent in Type 2 diabetes, perhaps only 10% or so after 20 years. These numbers are older figures; hopefully more patients are spared this in the modern era of better control, but you will still have days when you will feel swamped with proliferative concerns.

THE DISEASE

In macular edema, the problem stems from blood vessels that are leaky. In PDR, the problem stems from blood vessels that have simply died off. This starts in the periphery and gradually moves toward the center. The dead and dying retina then releases vasoproliferative factors that stimulate new blood vessels to grow (Figure 1).

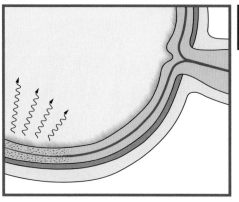

Figure 1. Ischemic peripheral retina emits vasoproliferative factors into the vitreous.

If the blood vessels simply grew in isolation, without any vitreous to latch onto, they would probably form beautiful branching patterns on the retinal surface—which would largely be of academic interest. Unfortunately, the vitreous is usually firmly attached to the retina in diabetics, and the blood vessels love to grow up into it like kudzu on a trellis (Figure 2).

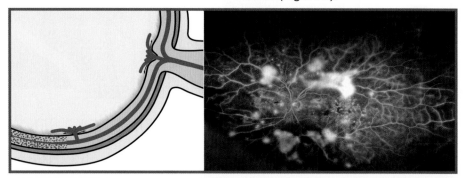

Figure 2. New vessels grow into the vitreous in response to the vasoproliferative substances. The photograph is a wide-field FA showing extensive peripheral capillary dropout and secondary neovascularization at the border of perfused and non-perfused retina. (Photo courtesy of Raj K. Maturi, M.D.)

All this would be bad enough, but it gets worse. These new blood vessels are quite leaky, and even if they don't hemorrhage, they allow serum components into the vitreous that the vitreous would normally never see. These compounds cause the vitreous to shrink up sooner than it otherwise would. Although vitreous collapse is a normal aging phenomenon, in proliferative retinopathy the contraction process is accelerated and tends to be more vicious. This is a real problem because the vitreous begins to pull on the new vessels (Figure 3).

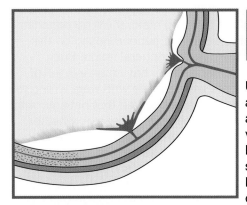

Figure 3. The vitreous contracts and starts to tug on the new vessels.

Unfortunately, the new vessels are now an extension of the retinal vasculature, and as such, they serve to lock the vitreous onto the retina wherever the blood vessels grow. This means that the shrinking vitreous now begins to tug on both the vessels and the retina. Moreover, connective tissue brought in by the new vessels also tends to shrink, which basically turns the vascular frond into the physiologic equivalent of a power winch that contracts in all directions. The result is that vessels at the surface of the retina are placed under constant tension, and the retina itself can be lifted from the pigment epithelium (Figure 4). If left untreated, the final result of this process is for the entire retina to be yanked off the back of the eye.

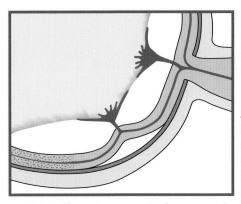

Figure 4. Progressive traction from the vitreous and the vessels begins to pull the retina off the RPE.

As this process is evolving, the stretched blood vessels crack open and bleed, subjecting the patient to periodic hemorrhages. The patient notices these hemorrhages as streaks, cobwebs and/ or clouds in their vision. This will usually motivate them to come in for an evaluation if they have been less than diligent in their follow up. Unfortunately, things are usually far advanced by the time the hemorrhages occur. The blood vessels will often be quite extensive and even if they can be controlled with laser, it is likely that there will still be a gradual buildup of traction as the vitreous and connective tissue continue to contract. Such traction may cause anything from mild metamorphopsia (from pulling gently on the posterior pole) to total vision loss (from a tractional retinal detachment). Intermediate problems can include anything from chronic macular edema (due to subtle traction on the macula) to insidious vision loss (from traction on the nerve). If the traction is very severe it may even rip holes in the retina. Once the vacuum-pack seal between the retina and retinal pigment epithelium is broken, the gliotic retina can snap off the back of the eye like a broken garage door spring. These are all Bad Things.

Back in the old days of retinopathy treatment, doctors would shoot at the growing blood vessels on the assumption that the blood vessels themselves were the root of the problem. It quickly became apparent that this approach was worse than useless. Treating the blood vessels alone tends to make them go bananas; they just get revved up by the irritation of the treatment superimposed on the powerful neovascular stimulus created by the dying peripheral retina. Such treatment did not address the more fundamental issue of having an eye full of vasoproliferative substances. Fortunately, there were people who were willing to think in a very open-minded fashion, and these folks observed that patients with lots of peripheral retinal scarring had less active proliferative disease, whether the scarring was from iatrogenic retinal treatment or preexisting ocular conditions. This eventually led them to try using a laser—or a xenon arc, or even focused light from the sun—to destroy the peripheral retina, shutting down the production of vasoproliferative factors and, in turn, shutting down the neovascularization. Apparently the thought of doing this was so counterintuitive that many people thought these pioneers were insane, but they were ultimately vindicated by the success of panretinal photocoagulation as demonstrated by the Diabetic Retinopathy Study. By the way, these last sentences are horribly inadequate to relay the immense effort on the part of the many individuals who have given us this incredible tool to prevent blindness. Every once in awhile, as your foot is racking up numbers on the laser counter, you should think about the broad shoulders upon which we are all standing as we treat diabetics with proliferative disease.

Hunting Down Nonproliferative and Proliferative Retinopathy in Your Patient

Your eternal goal is to try to stop the above chain of events at an early stage before the diabetes can sink too many of its fangs into the retina—before the vessels and fibrovascular tissue have spread all over the place. You should therefore become adept at identifying anything that even remotely suggests the impending arrival of proliferative disease. This means becoming familiar with the various stages of nonproliferative diabetic retinopathy (NPDR). Remember that NPDR can be minimal, mild, moderate or severe (Table 1 shows the standard classification scheme). Severe NPDR is of greatest importance, making it the one you need to be able to recognize unfailingly.

Fortunately, the 4-2-1 rule makes matters relatively easy when it comes to sorting out patients with good-bad retinopathy from those with bad-bad retinopathy. The 4-2-1 part refers to four quadrants of hemorrhages, two quadrants of venous beading or one quadrant of intraretinal microvascular abnormalities

(IRMAs). If a patient has any one of these criteria, then they have severe NPDR. The required amount for each of these findings is defined by the standard photographs used in all of the studies, and you should cram these images into your brain so that you can quickly pick out a patient at risk.

Table 1 / Classification of Diabetic Retinopathy

Level	Definition
Minimal nonproliferative retinopathy	Microaneurysms only
Mild nonproliferative retinopathy	Microaneurysms and one or more of the following: • Retinal hemorrhage • Hard exudates • Nerve fiber layer infarct
Moderate nonproliferative retinopathy	Hemorrhages and microaneurysms > standard photograph 2A in at least one quadrant and one or more of the following: • Nerve fiber layer infarct • Venous beading • Intraretinal microvascular abnormality
Severe nonproliferative retinopathy	One of the following: • Hemorrhages/microaneurysms > standard photograph 2A in all 4 quadrants • Venous beading in at least 2 quadrants • IRMA > standard photograph 8A
Proliferative retinopathy	Neovascularization on the disc or elsewhere
High-risk proliferative retinopathy	One or more of the following: • Neovascularization of the disc > 1/4 disc area • Any neovascularization of the disc and vitreous/preretinal hemorrhage • Neovascularization > 1/2 disc area with vitreous/preretinal hemorrhage
Advanced proliferative retinopathy	Proliferative retinopathy with tractional retinal detachment or with extensive vitreous hemorrhage

(Reproduced, with permission, from Fong DS, Ferris FL, Focal Points: Clinical Modules for Ophthalmologists, "Practical Management of Diabetic Retinopathy," American Academy of Ophthalmology, 2003.)

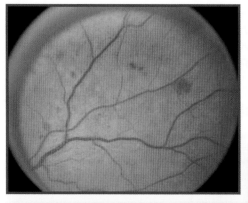

Figure 5. (Left) ETDRS Standard Photograph 2a, showing severe hemorrhages and microaneurysms (remember—you need these in four quadrants to get severe NPDR). (Courtesy of the Early Treatment Diabetic Retinopathy Study Group)

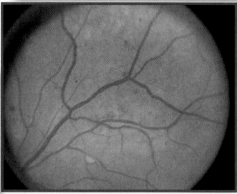

Figure 6. (Right) ETDRS Standard Photograph 6a, the criterion for going from mild to moderate venous beading. Notice that you don't need a lot. If you can see obvious venous beading in a patient, then it's bad (but you need two quadrants for severe NPDR). Also, be sure that it is venous beading and not just venous caliber changes. With true venous beading the beaded section must be wider than the normal caliber and because venous beading tends to be a late finding you should also judge it by the company it keeps—there should be other worrisome findings as well. (Courtesy of the Early Treatment Diabetic Retinopathy Study Group)

Figure 7. (Below) ETDRS Standard Photograph 8a. The circles show the odd, curlicue shape of IRMA. (Courtesy of the Early Treatment Diabetic Retinopathy Study Group)

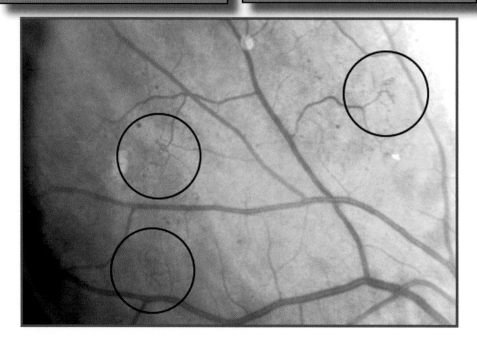

If memorizing the scheme is too painful, you can simplify it this way: if you look in and you can see obvious venous beading and/or definite IRMA, then the patient has severe NPDR or something very close to it. See the blue box if you think they have severe NPDR based on hemorrhages alone…

Although the presence of hemorrhages is one of the criteria for severe NPDR, as a practical matter it can be a less reliable predictor in clinical practice. Hemorrhages, like glory, can be fleeting, and they are not quite as dependable as hardcore venous beading and IRMA.[1] Just review the chapter on differential diagnosis to see the many ways hemorrhages may be unrelated to factors that cause proliferative disease. Then look in Chapter 16, where hemorrhages can resolve with institution of good systemic control. Finally, remember how patients on blood thinners may have very dramatic hemorrhages that have nothing to do with NPDR. The real point here is that if you think a patient has NPDR solely because of four quadrants of hemorrhages, and if you are going to treat them with laser, you should be sure they don't have hemorrhages for other reasons.

When it comes to hunting down evidence of severe NPDR, hemorrhages and venous beading tend to be fairly obvious. IRMAs, on the other hand, can be a bit trickier to identify. IRMAs are tiny, and are usually located in little patches outside the arcades, so it is something that you have to look for with your 90-diopter lens (or 78-diopter or whatever fundus-o-rama lens is being marketed this year by the lens manufacturers). You will need to have the patient look in different directions, similar to the indirect ophthalmoscope exam, and you will need to perfect your ability to use an indirect slit lamp lens for this purpose—something that has to be mastered in order to do a thorough exam for diabetic retinopathy.

Late-Seventies programmed-learning moment: What is a skill that has to be mastered in order to do a thorough exam for diabetic retinopathy?

    a. Understanding the conoid of Sturm
    b. Understanding phacodynamics
    c. Understanding Medicare
    d. Using a slit lamp indirect lens to study the midperiphery
    e. Do you see why the Seventies were so much fun?

It is really hard to manage diabetics without being able to do this.

When hunting for IRMAs you are looking for fine, irregular vessels that seem to be within or just at the surface of the retina—they do not follow any normal flow pattern and tend to meander around in a tiny area. Sadly, almost every attempt to reproduce photos of IRMAs is foiled by the limitations of the printing process—Figure 8 is a blowup of the standard ETDRS figure, so you get some idea of what you are looking for.

Why bother with this? Eyes with severe NPDR have as much as a 50% chance of developing some degree of PDR within one year, and perhaps a 15% chance of developing high-risk PDR. These averages are from the ETDRS—your mileage may vary with specific patients. If a patient has a long history of good control and very slow progression of their retinopathy, then their risk is much less. If they have poor control and are rapidly going to severe NPDR, then they are far more likely to get into trouble. The point is that knowing the stages of NPDR allows you to determine the patient's risk for progression to PDR and to decide how closely to follow the patient. Staging the patient may also help you decide whether they need panretinal photocoagulation before they get a chance to develop proliferative disease. Vide infra.

WHICH BRINGS US TO PDR Itself...

Although severe NPDR may be the ideal time to identify potential for trouble, proliferative diabetic retinopathy is your true enemy. Fortunately, PDR does not tend to be subtle. Even very small neovascularization at the disc (NVD) is readily apparent, simply because the vessels weave over the nerve in a path very different from the normal radial capillaries. Remember that NVD does not really need to be exclusively at the disc to be called NVD—vessels within 1 disc diameter of the nerve also qualify.

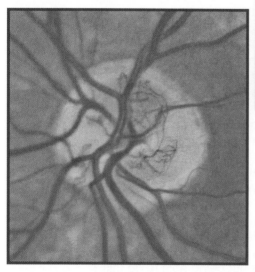

Figure 8. This is the picture that launched a million lasers. It is Standard Photograph 10a from the Arlie House Classification System—and it shows the size of NVD that qualifies as high-risk. (Courtesy of the Early Treatment Diabetic Retinopathy Study Group)

Neovascularization located further from the disc (known as neovascularization elsewhere—NVE) can sometimes be fainter, and can therefore be difficult to distinguish from IRMA if it is small. IRMA is localized within the retina, and although it may be irregular, it usually does not have a latticework of blood vessels as one sees with neovascularization. NVE is on top of the retina; sometimes it is flat and grows along the surface, while sometimes it is elevated and grows up into the vitreous. A fluorescein angiogram (FA) is helpful for determining the difference in problematic cases; IRMA may leak a bit, but it doesn't leak anywhere near as much as true neovascularization.

On the other hand, an FA will light up small patches of neo like a Broadway marquee. Ideally, you should not need an FA to identify even very early neo—you should have found it with a careful exam of the periphery as discussed above. If the view is hazy, though, or if you are still not sure whether there is any neo present, an FA can be very helpful (Figure 11).

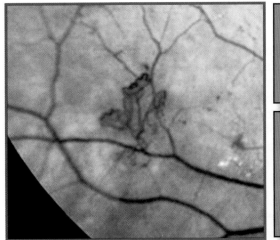

Figure 9. (Left) A typical small patch of NVE. Note how it consists of multiple branching vessels. If you could see it in stereo, you would note that it is growing off the surface of the retina into the vitreous.

Figure 10. (Below) The circles highlight patches of IRMA that are obvious on the red free on the left, but barely leak dye in the later phase of the angiogram on the right. Compare this to the profuse leakage that occurs with true neovascularization (e.g., Figure 11).

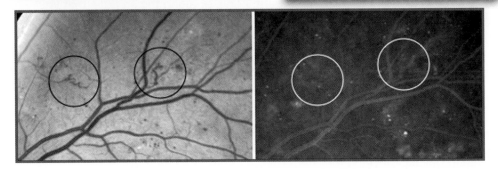

Figure 11 is also notable because it shows a type of retinopathy that can be very deceptive unless you look carefully. Some patients will have what is known as a "featureless retina." This means that the usual signs of disease, such as multiple hemorrhages, are no longer present, presumably because the retina has just plain died off. You will miss the early proliferative disease in these cases if you just quickly screen the fundus with a 20D lens and do not study the retina at the slit lamp.

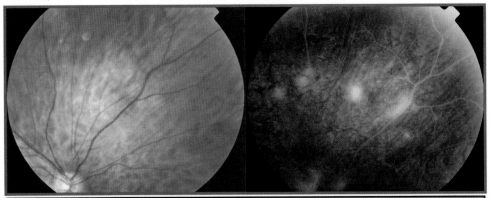

Figure 11. An example of how an angiogram can light up NVE that is not especially visible on clinical exam. Although the color photo does not show the neo, it is likely that a careful 90D exam of the periphery would have identified the small new vessels. Also note that the color shows a very "featureless retina"—the retina is so damaged that the usual signs of worrisome retinopathy are absent; there are no telltale hemorrhages, etc.

Incidentally, if you are doing an FA to look for new vessels, be sure to spell out to the photographer what you are looking for so they will scan the periphery for anything that lights up. It is easy to focus only on the posterior pole when doing angiograms, but there is a lot of data in the periphery, especially with diabetes. It makes sense to routinely have your photographer do a survey of the periphery in the midphases to look for any significant leakage that indicates neovascularization. This will also give you an idea of how much capillary dropout there is in the periphery, and can sometimes help determine where you place your panretinal photocoagulation pattern. If nothing else, obtaining photos of the periphery will help your photographers to improve, and you will be less likely to miss whatever the periphery is trying to tell you.

> **By the way,** it is always a bit embarrassing to order an FA for macular edema, only to find buds of neo at the nerve or along the arcades that you didn't see because you were too busy studying the topology of the macula. Of course, it is even more embarrassing to completely miss the buds of neo on the FA and then spot them when you look at the angiogram three months later because the patient had a vitreous hemorrhage that you could have prevented. Been there, done that.
>
> Missing something obvious is much less likely at the early stages of your career, when everything is new and exciting. It is much more likely to happen when you have some experience and confidence and you begin to chug along quickly. Develop a systematic way to read an FA in order not to miss anything, and try to stick with it no matter how fast you want to go—it will save you again and again.

When it comes to sniffing out PDR, another important clue is the presence of some type of vitreous hemorrhage. A big hemorrhage is usually about as subtle as a golf cart in a hotel bathtub—the diagnosis is easy. Sometimes, though, patients will have the symptoms of a hemorrhage (i.e., dots, streaks, cobwebs and/or floaters in their vision) but there is no obvious blood on first inspection. Study such patients carefully. It is possible for patients to have limited hemorrhages, for which they will be very symptomatic, yet you will not see any blood because the amount is small or it has been rapidly washed out. Look at the vitreous with the slit lamp, as you would for a uveitis patient—sometimes the only heme to be found is a few red blood cells in the anterior vitreous. Also, carefully inspect the lower vitreous. Subtle hemorrhages will gravitate down there, and you may need to use a 90-diopter to find faint clouds of blood floating around. This is important, because if there is blood, you really have to look carefully for neovascularization—even get an FA, if necessary.

Diabetics can have hemorrhages without neo, though, so don't just look for "clouds of red" and then bust out the laser. First of all, diabetics tend to have a stickier vitreous that doesn't separate as easily. If they do get even a partial age-related vitreous detachment, all of the fragile capillaries on the retinal surface are more likely to bleed as the vitreous peels away. This can create a transient hemorrhage but this does not represent an ongoing threat to the patient's vision so no treatment is needed. This partly explains why there was a whole subset of patients in the Diabetic Retinopathy Study who fell into the category of having a vitreous hemorrhage without obvious PDR and why many of these patients did not need any laser (more on this below).

By the way, never forget that diabetics can get non-diabetic problems, such as retinal tears. If a vitreous hemorrhage makes you go into proliferative-disease hunter-killer mode, you can totally miss a tear if you don't also remember to study the far periphery for new breaks. Just try to keep an open mind about all the wonderful ways an eye can go bad and do not limit your thinking to diabetic complications just because a patient is diabetic.

> **Patients** who present several months after their symptoms began can also be confusing, because older hemorrhages can decolorize and look like whitish or yellowish globs at the bottom of the vitreous cavity (so-called "chicken fat" hemorrhages). Do not mistake these old hemorrhages for inflammatory vitreous changes such as snowballs or snow banking. Bombing a hemorrhagic diabetic eye with steroids is bad for the patient—and will remove additional points from your god-of-ophthalmology score.

PUTTING IT ALL TOGETHER

OK, so now you have scoured the fundus for signs of IRMA or early PDR. Exactly why do you need to memorize the 4-2-1 rule and hunt around for all this stuff, anyway?

There is no question that one of the landmark studies in all of ophthalmology was the Diabetic Retinopathy Study (DRS), which clearly demonstrated the usefulness of laser treatment in avoiding blindness back in the 1970s.[2] (Both the DRS and the ETDRS produced a host of papers; the cited reference is an example.)

As part of this study, proliferative diabetic retinopathy was classified into low-risk and high-risk disease. (Nowadays "low-risk" PDR is called PDR without high-risk characteristics—see Table 1.) Determining whether a patient has high-risk PDR involves adding up various factors to assign the level of disease. For instance, high-risk vessels at the disc had to be at least one-quarter to one-third disc area (Figure 8 is the standard example chosen for this), and NVE was considered to be significant if it was greater than one-half disc area. Table 2 (on the next page) shows a good summary of how all the different factors were added up to assign the overall risk. For those of us not employed as biostatisticians, however, each one of the following is an admittedly less elegant but simpler approximation for how to call high-risk PDR:

1: Any NVD that you can easily see is high-risk PDR.
2: Pre-retinal or vitreous blood in the eye with new vessels anywhere is high-risk PDR. 'Nuff said.

Table 2 / Definition of High Risk PDR

High-risk PDR was defined as any one of following:

- mild neovascularization of the disc (NVD) with vitreous hemorrhage
- moderate to severe NVD with or without vitreous hemorrhage (> or = Standard 10A, showing 1/4 to 1/3 disc area of NVD)
- moderate (1/2 disc area) neovascularization elsewhere (NVE) with vitreous hemorrhage

High-risk PDR was also defined by any combination of three of the four retinopathy risk factors:

- presence of vitreous or preretinal hemorrhage
- presence of new vessels
- location of new vessels on or near the optic disc
- moderate to severe extent of new vessels

(American Academy of Ophthalmology, Basic and Clinical Science Course, Section 12, Retina and Vitreous 2007-2008 page 109.)

Once you decide a patient has high-risk PDR, you are obligated to treat with panretinal photocoagulation. The reason is that patients tend to do rather horribly on their own once they have reached high-risk disease. In the DRS, treatment cut the risk of severe vision loss by about 50% over the course of the study—and that was at a time when diabetics were not as well controlled medically, and the treatment was often hammered in all at once (and was therefore more likely to decrease the vision). It is likely that these days we obtain even better results with staged treatment and more emphasis on better medical care. Figure 12 is the classic graph of the overall results.

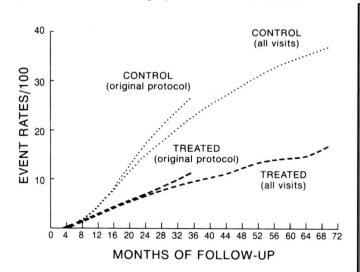

Figure 12. Cumulative rates of severe visual loss for the DRS (the protocol was changed in 1976 to allow more treatment of high-risk eyes). This graph, and the heroic work behind its discovery, is truly awesome (in the traditional, non-surfer sense of the word). (The Diabetic Retinopathy Study Research Group, DRS report no. 8, Ophthalmology 1981; 88: 583-600, Copyright Elsevier 1981.)

But deciding to treat definite high-risk proliferative disease is the easy part. The hard part is deciding about treatment in situations that are less black and white...

DRS/ETDRS GAMES When to Do Premature Photocoagulation

Although the DRS clearly demonstrated the need for treatment in patients with high-risk disease, no one was sure how aggressive to be in patients with less than high-risk disease. One aspect of the ETDRS looked at this and found a trend suggesting a beneficial treatment effect if patients were given PRPs at any level of nonproliferative diabetic retinopathy (NPDR).[3] However, the treatment benefits were very small with earlier levels of NPDR. For instance, there was only a dinky subset of patients with mild or moderate NPDR who seemed to benefit from early treatment. Because PRP has definite risks (which will be discussed at length in the upcoming chapters), it is felt that observation is best for these patients.

When the retinopathy progresses to severe NPDR or PDR without high-risk characteristics, it turns out that the treatment benefit was more pronounced— but still fairly small. As a result, the same conservative approach generally applies: Given the hassle and risk of treatment and relatively small benefit, these patients, especially Type 1 diabetics, may be better off with careful observation rather than laser. There are, however, other factors that may make you decide to treat such patients. Here are some:

1. Severe progressive disease in the fellow eye. Diabetic eyes tend to head down the same path, and the first eye will let you know what the second eye may decide to do.

2. The patient's ability to follow up. This may be a very important factor in developing countries, where logistics and economics may prevent careful sequential evaluations, and where early treatment may give a patient much better odds of remaining a functioning member of society.

3. Poor control and/or lots of medical problems may warrant earlier intervention, since these patients may go downhill faster and/or may miss appointments.

4. A patient who needs to be on Coumadin may need earlier treatment, given the risk of more pronounced bleeding if more advanced proliferative disease is allowed to develop.

5. A very important factor is the rate of change of the patient's disease. A patient who has good control and has smoldered along with mild to moderate NPDR can easily be monitored if they slowly begin to develop severe NPDR or low-risk PDR. On the other hand, a patient who is rapidly going through these stages is at much greater risk for rapid progression to high-risk disease, and should have earlier treatment. (Incidentally, the ability to understand terms like "the rate of change" justifies those calculus classes you took years ago. They were worth it.)

6. The type of diabetes also plays a role. A later analysis of the data suggested that patients with Type 2 diabetes, or patients older than 40 years old (which is usually the same thing), are more likely to benefit from scatter photocoagulation when they have severe NPDR or early PDR without high-risk characteristics. This did not seem to be true for patients with Type 1 diabetes who had the same degree of retinopathy. It is not clear why this is the case; perhaps older patients are more likely to get a vitreous hemorrhage once they get neo because their vitreous is more jiggly. Whatever the reason, this does data support consideration of earlier treatment in older patients.[4]

What if there is a vitreous hemorrhage but no obvious neo?

Although knowing when to intervene earlier is important, it is also good to know when to hold off. Such a situation may occur when you are faced with a patient who has a vitreous hemorrhage but no evidence of neovascularization. The DRS showed that a vitreous hemorrhage alone is generally not an indication for PRP, but this is true only if you are certain there is no neovascularization. If there is a localized preretinal hemorrhage that blocks the view of a section of the retina, or a dense vitreous hemorrhage that allows only a limited view, it is usually best to assume there are new blood vessels somewhere and treat the patient.

> **Remember** that if the hemorrhage is so dense that there is no view, you have to get an ultrasound to be sure the retina is not being pulled off. You are taking a big risk for both yourself and your patient if you can't see the retina and you don't get an ultrasound; if something is going wrong back there, it is usually bad to do nothing.

The nature of the retinopathy in the fellow eye can help in such a situation, too. If the fellow eye has already had proliferative disease that required laser, it is worthwhile considering laser in the second eye even if you do not see any obvious neovascularization. On the other hand, if there is only minimal diabetic disease in the fellow eye, observation may be the best course.

If the hemorrhage is mild, though, you need to study the retinal periphery carefully, or even consider fluorescein angiography to help you decide whether there are new vessels. If there are no vessels, then it is definitely better to watch such patients; recall that the diabetic vitreous is sticky and is more likely to break a few capillaries if it separates. You will end up needlessly burning retina if you automatically treat every diabetic with a mild vitreous hemorrhage.

Finally, for the second time in the same chapter, never forget that diabetics can get non-diabetic problems such as retinal tears, so remember to inspect the far periphery closely—don't just look in the mid-periphery and quit if you don't see anything.

What if a patient shows up with old, burned-out disease that was never treated?

Although most of your life you will be faced with patients who are in the progressive stages of PDR, remember that if left untreated the neovascular stimulus eventually fades as the retina just plain dies off. Most of the time, if the disease is allowed to run its course the retina ends up like a shriveled orchid in the center of a blind eye (hence the existence of books such as this one). You may, however, occasionally see patients in whom this process has occurred with little disruption of the central retina—these patients essentially avoided the typical disastrous outcome and "survived" the proliferative phase of their retinopathy. Such patients often have very broad areas of fibrosis in the periphery, where the old neovascularization involuted and became quiescent. Deciding whether to treat such patients can be difficult—the standard rules do not apply. These patients have somehow achieved a metastable state, and there is always a concern that by going in and aggressively treating with laser you will push them into hemorrhagic or tractional problems that they might not otherwise have developed. In general, however, it is safer to gently work in a PRP, rather than to do nothing. This is because the wide swathes of untreated peripheral retina may become more ischemic with time, and lead to late problems such as recurrent retinal proliferation or anterior segment neovascularization.

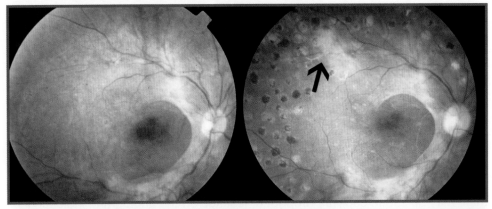

Figure 13. A patient with fibrotic, end-stage PDR. Note how everything seems to be quiescent prior to treatment, but after laser, there is an area where subtle neovascularization regressed and became fibrotic (arrow). The omnipresent neovascular stimulus of the ischemic retina makes treatment a safer bet than observation in eyes like this; you are buying the patient insurance that nothing worse happens in the future. Do go slow if you treat such an eye, however. Rapid carpet-bomb laser will likely stir things up in such a fragile eye, perhaps even causing a tractional retinal detachment.

If you decide to treat an eye like this, and usually you will, the patient (and you) must understand that there is always a small risk of stirring up trouble. The one thing you don't want to do is to decide that you have to make up for lost time by hammering the entire retina aggressively. This carries a high risk of screwing things up in such a delicate eye. It is much better to treat these patients gradually over a number of sessions, and to avoid heavy burns around the atrophic or tractionally detached retina which could lead to hole formation.

Do you have to have an FA before a PRP? No. But...

An FA is not mandatory before treating isolated PDR. The great ophthalmic court in the sky should not frown upon you if you do not get one, especially because in many places it may not be an option. However, if it is available, you should consider doing the test for a few reasons:

1. An FA can give you an idea of exactly where most of the capillary ischemia is in the periphery; this will help you assess how bad the disease is, where to treat, and how aggressive you will need to be with your PRP (Figure 14).

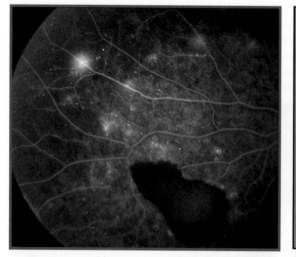

Figure 14. Another example of an FA lighting up neovascularization and defining the border between perfused and non-perfused retina. Note the preretinal hemorrhage that does not appear to be near the obvious new vessels. There may be neovascularization underneath the heme, or it may have originated from puffy and swollen vessels inside the perfused retina that are just beginning to sprout new vascular channels.

2. You will get info about the functional status of the macular blood vessels. Sometimes the macula can look fairly decent on clinical exam and OCT, but there may be subtle capillary dropout or leakage on the angiogram, indicating that the macula is more fragile than you would think. These findings suggest that you should go *very* slowly when you start doing the PRP to avoid stressing out the capillaries and making the patient's central vision worse due to macular edema. Also, if the patient is beginning to develop capillary dropout in the temporal macula you will need to warn the patient about the potential for vision loss that exists with even successful treatment of their proliferative disease. In the manly world of retina specialists, where manly men and women think up manly names for microscopic problems in order to feel more manly, this particular pattern is sometimes called the flying wedge of death (Figure 15). This pattern does not

always progress, and in fact, some patients may be stable for years—especially if they have good control. Still, it is important to let the patient know what you are worried about and what it might mean to their vision.

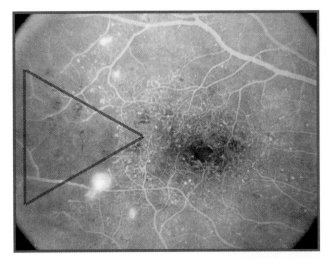

Figure 15. A triangular wedge of ischemia encroaching into the macula.

3. A less "medically necessary" but remarkably powerful use of the angiogram is for patient education. If a patient has yet to display symptoms of their retinopathy, you can try to convince them of the impending danger by showing them the fronds of neovascularization surrounding their posterior pole. This is not a reason to subject a patient to an invasive test like an FA, but if a study is done, it is a shame to not use it for this purpose.

On the other hand (and the problem with being a conscientious doctor is recognizing that there is always an "other hand"), you may find yourself in a practice where obtaining an angiogram is not a simple thing. If you do not have easy access to an FA, it may be better to go without one if your clinical sense is that the retina does not hold any big surprises. Making the patient jump through hoops to undergo the pleasure of an FA, and to get even more medical bills, may be enough to drive them away from being treated. This is way worse than not having an FA in the first place. Everything is a balance...

References and Suggested Reading

1.   Wilkinson CP, Ferris FL, 3rd, Klein RE, et al. Proposed international clinical diabetic retinopathy and diabetic macular edema disease severity scales. Ophthalmology 2003;110:1677-82.

2.   Photocoagulation treatment of proliferative diabetic retinopathy. Clinical application of Diabetic Retinopathy Study (DRS) findings, DRS Report Number 8. The Diabetic Retinopathy Study Research Group. Ophthalmology 1981;88:583-600.

3.   Early photocoagulation for diabetic retinopathy. ETDRS report number 9. Early Treatment Diabetic Retinopathy Study Research Group. Ophthalmology 1991;98:766-85.

4.   Ferris F. Early photocoagulation in patients with either type I or type II diabetes. Trans Am Ophthalmol Soc 1996;94:505-37.

Davis MD, Blodi BA. Proliferative Diabetic Retinopathy. In: Ryan SJ. Retina, 4th ed. Philadelphia: Elsevier Mosby, 2006:v.2, pp 1285-1322.

Folk JC, Pulido JS. Laser photocoagulation of the retina and choroid. San Francisco: American Academy of Ophthalmology, 1997.

Basic and Clinical Science Course Section 12: Retina and Vitreous. San Francisco: American Academy of Ophthalmology, 2008:pp109-132.

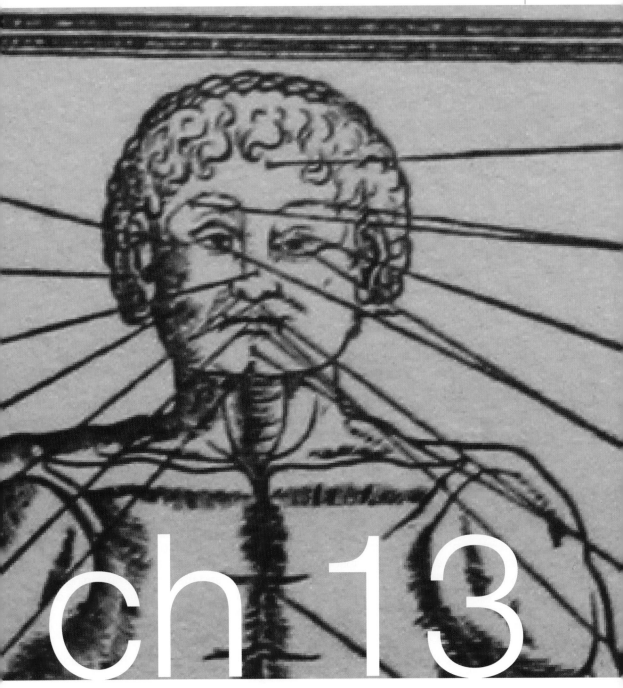

ch 13

Trust Me, I'm a Doctor PART TWO: The Informed Consent
for Panretinal Photocoagulation (PRP)

THE INFORMED CONSENT for Panretinal Photocoagulation (PRP)

Although the mechanics of doing a PRP can be daunting—and will be covered at length in the next chapter—perhaps the most difficult aspect of performing this procedure involves the informed consent. It can be very hard to provide an effective informed consent that gives the patient a fighting chance of actually understanding what on earth you are about to do to them. The general principles discussed in the section on informed consent for diabetic macular edema also apply here. However, a PRP is much more intense, and the results of treatment are even more likely to confuse the patient, so this chapter will emphasize points specific to doing a PRP.

THE DISEASE

As with macular edema, you have to start by educating the patient about the nature of the disease. This is easy if you have a sophisticated patient who has already read an entire retina textbook on the internet. If you have such a carriage-trade practice, with nothing but wealthy, educated patients, you don't even need to read this section—just tell them about the pathophysiology of retinopathy and the complications and you are done.

For those who practice in the real world, though, recognize that the nuances of proliferative retinopathy can be quite confusing to patients. So you might as well start with the basics, and this includes pointing out the irreplaceable nature of the retina. (You will find patients that truly believe that they will be able to get a total eye transplant if your laser doesn't work. Really. Educate them about this right at the start, so they are not surprised later—it will also help motivate them to take better care of themselves.)

Next, you need to relay the relentless (and asymptomatic) way that diabetes kills off the distal retinal blood vessels, which in turn causes ischemia and the generation of vasoproliferative factors, which in turn causes bad blood vessels and bleeding, etc., etc. The absolute key is to inform them that the goal of the laser is to get rid of these vasoproliferative factors, and that you are *not* going to "laser their blood vessels." It is very difficult to convey the "indirect" nature of this treatment, but the importance of making sure they understand this cannot be stressed enough.

First of all, if patients think you are simply going in and cauterizing the bad blood vessels, they will assume—if they hemorrhage subsequent to the laser—that you must have failed in your task. It is hard enough taking care of diabetics as it is—you don't want them thinking you are incompetent for the wrong reasons.

Second, if they can really understand that the goal is to eliminate the bad chemicals, and that only then will the bad blood vessels start to shrink, they then may be able to understand why they can have hemorrhages even after multiple laser sessions: The blood vessels may not completely disappear in spite of treatment because the laser can only indirectly convince them to go away. It also helps patients to understand why the problem can be controlled for a period of time, but then it can come back. In this case more of their peripheral retina dies off over time and there is a renewed stimulus for vascular growth. As a result, even more laser is required to control the problem.

You have to take the explanation a bit further, though, because some patients will still have hemorrhages with maximal laser. Explain that some of the new vessels can be stuck to the vitreous, and as the vitreous contracts, it can pull at the blood vessels, resulting in recurrent bleeding. This becomes a mechanical problem that no amount of laser can control. The management of this problem is discussed in the chapter on referral for vitrectomy, but this concept has to be conveyed to the PRP patient so they can understand the limits of the laser and why they may still have problems.

Successfully conveying all of the above is way harder than doing the stupid treatment. You really need to drive home the point that you will be doing every-thing you can to control things, but in some ways treating proliferative retinopa-thy is like making a bed with a 30-foot pole—you can push things in the right direction but it is not clear how well everything will end up.

And this is only the beginning of a complete discussion with the patient...

For instance, depending on the situation there are variations to the consent. The touchiest presentation is if the patient has disease that needs treatment but they have never had any symptoms. You have nowhere to go but *down* in this case, and education is crucial. Having an angiogram is helpful, because you can at least show them the massive leaking thunderheads of neovascularization that are building up on the horizon of their vision. These patients really need to understand where they are headed without treatment, i.e., severe, permanent vision loss, and they need to understand that the laser does not completely eliminate the risk of transient hemorrhages or gradual blurring over time, though it will very likely allow them to avoid blindness.

Occasional patients will have an annoying problem that is especially bad if you are treating them before they have symptoms: As the new vessels begin to contract from the PRP, they can hemorrhage. In other words, you start with an asymptomatic patient, and a week or two after their first laser they get their first vitreous hemorrhage (which can be truly frightening—these people have been living in dread of both blindness and other complications of their disease; see Chapter 20). If you haven't prepared them for this type of hemorrhage, you may lose the patient to follow up. This would not be so bad if they then just went to someone else; you would deserve to lose patients for being so obtuse. However, the usual pattern is for them to wander off after such a hemorrhage thinking that all doctors and lasers are crazy and they don't follow up with anyone. They then show up a year or two later with really awful disease that may not be fixable. The point is that treating diabetes is like three-dimensional chess: You have to be able to anticipate not only what the disease might do to the patient, but also what the disease might do after you try to treat it; and then you especially need to anticipate the patient's emotional response to all of this. You may be the best laserist in the world, but if you do not prepare them in advance for hemorrhages and thereby lose the patient's trust, you will end up being the worst laserist in the world.

Another problem occurs when patients show up late in the game with a lot of neovascular tissue. Such patients usually have had at least a few symptoms, but often the symptoms do not give them any idea how bad the situation really is. You have to prepare these patients for a real rollercoaster ride. First of all, any patient with severe disease will usually have intermittent hemorrhaging in spite of laser—big vascular fronds just do not give up without a fight. In addition, any patient who has a great deal of neovascular tissue will inevitably develop tractional forces from the fibroblasts that ride along with the vessels. These forces tend to show up several months after your laser. They may be mild, but with advanced proliferative disease they are usually strong enough to create metamorphopsia, or even a tractional retinal detachment involving the posterior pole. It is important to give the patient advance warning about this. Then if they do need a vitrectomy they are prepared for the possibility and realize that it is a consequence of their proliferative disease and not your laser.

The point is that whatever degree of proliferative retinopathy they have, you have to warn them that things may get darker before the dawn. If you start laser-ing them without really drilling this possibility into their heads, you can imagine the charitable thoughts they will have about you as you try to explain the above problems after the fact. Then just imagine what they will think if they go on to get tractional problems with permanent changes in their vision—or even if they have a little bit of vitreous haze from a hemorrhage that never completely clears. You will be congratulating yourself on having avoided severe blindness while they are remembering how great they could see before you started lasering them. Welcome to the fundamental patient-doctor disparity in the world of retina—we can be screamingly happy and they think we are monsters. Constant repetition of the nature of the problem and the potential for trouble—even with successful treatment—is your only hope of having the patient at least partially on your side.

Finally, they need to understand something about the time frame of treating proliferative disease. If they have mild disease that you are treating preemptively this is not much of an issue because usually you will treat them and save them and nothing much happens. The time frame is much more of an issue if they have aggressive disease with active hemorrhaging, or if they have big vessels that are likely to hemorrhage and/or scar up. Proliferative disease like this does tend to eventually burn out—but it usually takes a year or two for things to really settle down.

Of course, this does not mean that they can mark their calendar and assume that in two years they will be done—even burned-out retinopathy needs long-term monitoring and occasional tweaks. This also assumes that their disease is not rampant and that the patient is religious about their follow up and their systemic control. (If they have bad disease the battle can go on forever but this is usually something that your friendly neighborhood retina specialist will need to deal with, not you.) They need to understand that they are beginning a long-term process and although there is usually light at the end of the tunnel it takes a lot of time and effort to get there.

So—all of the above covers what might happen if things go right. What if things go wrong?

COMPLICATIONS

This is an annoying area to bring up, because you can spin an exhaustive tale about the nature of the disease and the importance of PRP, but once you mention that the laser can make things worse, you can pretty much assume that it is the *only* thing the patient and family will remember. Hopefully by following the teachings of your mentors, and from your own experience, you will be able to treat these patients with only minimal side effects. Still, there is that chance that they could sit back from your laser and be permanently worse—and you cannot avoid discussing this. The actual means by which vision can worsen is discussed at length in Chapter 16—your job is to cover the possibilities in the consent, but never ever have to actually deal with them.

To start with, even if you don't have a true complication there are potential nuisances that patients my notice after a PRP that they need to be informed about. For instance, some patients may notice changes in their side vision, night vision, focusing ability, and increased glare symptoms. If they have already had a hemorrhage, they won't mind these things too much because, like Ebenezer Scrooge meeting the Ghost of Christmas Future, they have had a taste of what is coming and they tend to view things like needing reading glasses in the proper perspective.

However, if you happen to be treating them prior to their having had any symptoms, and if they develop some of these problems, they will think you are an idiot. They were doing fine before you started lasering them, and now look at the mess you have gotten them into: reading glasses, sunglasses, night driving trouble, etc. You have to prepare them for these side effects, and you have to repeat the rationale for treatment at every laser to remind them what would happen without treatment. If you have done a careful informed consent, the patient will understand the need to be treated, and they will stick with you. Fortunately, with careful treatment you can usually avoid inducing these side effects, but you never want anything to come as a surprise to a patient.

It is also worth mentioning that the above problems cannot be blamed entirely on the laser—they are also part of having a sick diabetic eye. In other words, symptoms like changes in side vision, night vision, focusing ability, and resistance to glare are also part of what happens when most of the retina is slowly suffocating due to diabetes. It is one of the great ironies that by discussing these potential side effects of a PRP you have pretty much guaranteed that if they ever have these symptoms, they will blame your laser—even if the laser saved them and even if the laser is only partly responsible for the symptoms. This is why communication and repetition are so important when it comes to treating diabetics. Patients can easily draw unfair conclusions, and you have to anticipate this to keep them from wandering off and getting lost to follow up.

Also, remember that other doctors may look in your patient's eye and demonstrate their examination skills by saying something useful like, "Gee, you would not believe all the laser scars you have in the back of that eye!" (Review Chapter 5 for a full discussion on this.) Even if the patient does not have such an experience, they still tend to imagine that your PRP is gradually steamrolling away all of their retina, so you need to make sure they understand that your treatment is well away from the center of their vision, and that you are treating dead and dying retina that is good for nothing but poisoning the eye.

Finally, when discussing complications, remember to point out that the most feared "complication" is that the laser just plain does not stop their retinopathy, in which case they will definitely get worse—not from the laser, but from the disease.

Wrapping things up so we can get on to toasting retina in the next chapter...

Once again, this is all a lot of information. Recognize that patients often want to distill this—or any medical info—into very simple terms. Sometimes, these distillations can be shockingly unrelated to the carefully thought-out reality you have presented. For instance, upon hearing that there may be side effects of the laser, some patients will immediately choose to "take their risks with going blind from the diabetes as opposed to being made blind sooner with the laser." Usually, these thoughts are left unverbalized. If a patient seems unwilling to have treatment, or is poorly compliant, you need to specifically address these concerns by directly asking the patient what they are worried about.

Because understanding the rationale behind doing a PRP can be so counterintuitive, another crucial thing to do is to ask the patient to simply repeat back to you their understanding of what you have said. As discussed in Chapter 6, this a very powerful tool to make sure the patient is really thinking what you think the patient is thinking (which is hopefully somewhat close to what you are thinking).

> Don't forget that some patients will incorrectly conclude from your informed consent that they will inevitably go blind, and that the treatment only slows the process down. Watch for this and ask about it—patients can really mess themselves up if they get this into their head. Check back to Chapter 6 for a refresher if needed.

The PRP consent is a bit trickier than a macular edema consent, but the same general pattern applies: Cover the disease, cover the complications, cover the fact that the biggest problem is that the treatment may not stop it, and then talk about the mechanics of the treatment. Recognize that treating macular edema tends to result in smooth curves of response that are easier for the patient to understand—things get slowly better or they get slowly worse, and you do the best you can. Treating proliferative disease is much more of a stuttering, unpredictable mess, and you constantly need to anticipate not only everything that can go wrong, but also all the different ways the patient can misinterpret what is happening. Just keep repeating the information and listen carefully for indications that the patient is not getting it. Oh, and last but not least, never miss an opportunity to stress that the patient's systemic control plays a big role in how they respond to your laser. No matter how you do panretinal photocoagulation, it is still a very unpleasant experience and it can be a very powerful motivator if patients clearly understand that better control equals fewer PRPs.

"But Doc, I know somebody who was blinded by the laser…"

Recognize that panretinal photocoagulation is perhaps the most hated and feared treatment amongst diabetics, especially amongst less sophisticated patients. Many diabetics know someone who has been "blinded by the laser," and often it is a PRP that had something to do with it. If you are lucky, the patient will blurt out this concern and you can address it up front. If you are not lucky, you may get a vague sense of reluctance on the part of the patient—a sense that no matter how you try, you can't connect with them. If the patient does seem reluctant, you may need to specifically fish for this issue by asking whether the patient knows other people who have had laser treatment, and what their experiences were.

(Note: Another reason you may get this vague reluctance is because the patient has no money but does not want to talk about it—see Chapter 21 on The Big Bucks. A final reason the patient may be reluctant is that you are gradually turning into the jerk doctor you were always afraid you might become and everyone secretly hates and mistrusts you. You are on your own with this one.)

If this "blinded by the laser" issue does come up, it can be pointed out that usually any sense that the laser caused a problem is really due to the fact that the patient presented with severe disease and the laser simply could not control the process. In other words, the laser was too little, too late.

Here is a folksy story that might get the point across: Have the patient imagine that a train full of people is headed for a collapsed bridge, and the brakes are broken, so everyone is going to die. Well, suppose that some enterprising soul grabs a big safe, ties it to the train with a big rope, and then throws it out the door to try to slow down the train. The rope breaks and it doesn't work, and the train goes off the cliff. No one would blame the guy who threw out the safe for the fact that the train went off the cliff—it was just a desperate attempt to avoid a catastrophe. Then explain that the doctor who treated the person who "went blind from the laser" was just like the guy with the safe—it is not that the laser caused the blindness, but just that the laser couldn't stop it. Sometimes a parable like this can play big in the laser room.

Unfortunately, as discussed in the next chapters, panretinal photocoagulation is perhaps the one laser that is capable of blinding someone, so you cannot glibly blow off a concern like this with only a parable. Sometimes you can alleviate anxiety by getting more details about this "blinding laser." It may have been a completely different laser—for instance, there was an older treatment for macular degeneration that did indeed blind people by lasering away their fovea (but it was usually better than doing nothing). Still, it is possible that your patient's friend actually had a poorly done PRP. If it sounds like this was the case, all you can really do is point out that you will do everything possible to avoid such a problem. Go slowly with this—you have to be sure you are getting through.

Incidentally, you probably will not be able to tell whether any given "blinded by the laser" story represents a bad PRP or progression of disease in spite of a PRP. Heck, you probably won't even be able to tell whether it was something totally different, like maybe a diopter of astigmatism after Lasik (oh no!). Ultimately, it doesn't make any difference what happened; your goal is to provide a careful informed consent that covers all possibilities, so your patient will recognize that *you* recognize their concerns and that you are addressing them. You do not want to remotely suggest that their friend, relative, etc. was given a hatchet job of a laser. You were not there, and you do not have any idea about what really happened, so just focus on what you are trying to convey to your patient about their disease and their treatment.

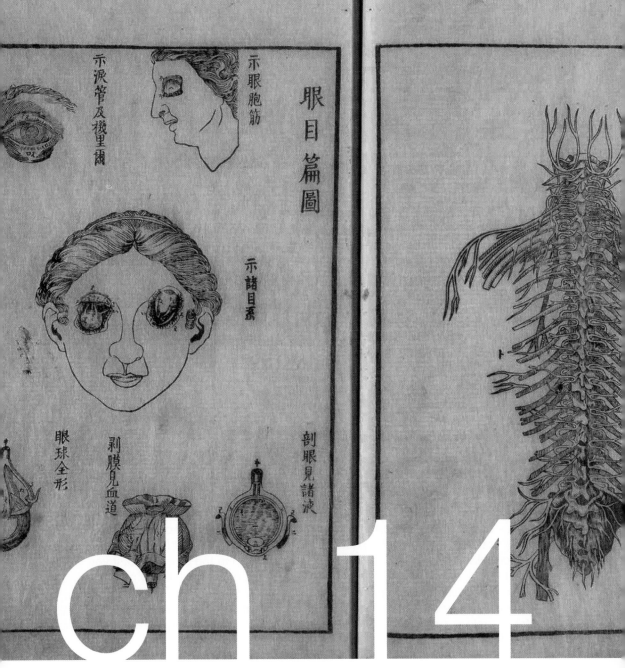

ch 14
Actually Doing Panretinal Photocoagulation (PRP)

Performing a PRP is one of those things that seems incredibly simple in the abstract, but actually requires a great deal of finesse to do properly. It is not just a matter of developing the technical skills needed to do the laser. You also have to consider the status of the eye and the systemic medical status of the patient. You even need to take into account far more subjective factors, such as the visual requirements of the patient and even their emotional status.

Back in the Seventies, the original Diabetic Retinopathy Study (DRS) called for a PRP to consist of 1200 to 1600 spots that were 500 to 1000 microns in size at the retina. These were to be placed approximately one-half burn width apart, from the arcades on out. This is a lot of laser. Because such treatment is the traditional standard, one would not be faulted if one ignored the rest of this chapter and just did this to every diabetic that needs a PRP—it is classic treatment from a classic paper. However, it is unlikely you are doing the type of cataract surgery they did back then, so perhaps it is worth looking deeper into why we do what we do…

First, Grasshopper, you must wrap your head around the fundamental contradiction inherent in doing a PRP. It can best be summarized in the following koan:

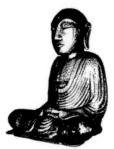
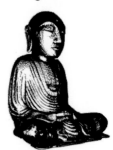

The best PRP is the worst PRP.

Studies have shown that a powerful, dense PRP gives one the best chance of long-term success. Unfortunately, it also gives one the best chance of having very noticeable side effects: decreased vision, loss of visual field, loss of night vision, glare, etc. The best PRP is the worst PRP. On the other hand, if you go light you are likely to avoid these complications, or they will be so mild that they do not interfere with the patient's life. (For instance, they may be much safer drivers—never underestimate the significance of your treatment decisions). Unfortunately, a safer, milder PRP carries a greater risk of problems with recurrent proliferative disease. The best PRP is the worst PRP.

Let's explore this a bit more. If you dig into the ETDRS and the DRS, you will realize that they led to numerous papers looking at all kinds of obscure things. Buried deep in two of these papers are some really useful graphs.[1, 2] They are reproduced here in their original pre-Microsoft Office glory. They show that the denser the treatment, the more likely it is that patients will avoid severe vision loss. You always need to remember these graphs if you decide to treat less than the standard DRS treatment.

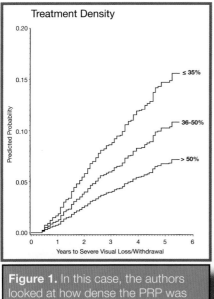

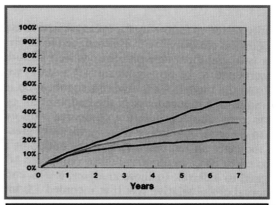

Figure 1. In this case, the authors looked at how dense the PRP was in peripheral photographs versus the probability of severe vision loss. The greater the density, the better the treatment worked (>50% treatment density was best). (Kaufman SC, Ferris FL, 3rd, Seigel DG, Davis MD, DeMets DL. Factors associated with visual outcome after photocoagulation for diabetic retinopathy. Diabetic Retinopathy Study Report #13. Invest Ophthalmol Vis Sci 1989;30:23-8.)

Figure 2. This was an arm of the ETDRS in which patients were assigned to no treatment (black), mild scatter PRP (orange), or standard PRP (dark red). They started with moderate to severe NPDR or low-risk PDR, and the y axis shows the probability of developing high-risk PDR. Stronger treatment resulted in much less risk of progression. (Figure 4 is a photo of the standard laser pattern and Figure 5 shows the mild pattern.) This graph was scanned from the original paper; note that you can actually see the print from the page behind it. Talk about ancient history... (Early Treatment Diabetic Retinopathy Study Research Group. Early photocoagulation for diabetic retinopathy, ETDRS Report #9. Ophthalmology, 1991;98:766-85. Copyright Elsevier.)

However, as Chapter 16 will be showing you, you can cause a world of hurt if you just give everyone a full-blown PRP. Also, remember that the graphs essentially represent dose-response curves, and as with any drug, you do not automatically give the highest dose to everyone just because it seems to work best when you look at the entire population. As a physician, your job is to pick the right dose for each individual patient. You will find that many patients will do quite well with less than a full dose of laser. Or, to look at it another way, you are trying to use the lowest dose of laser necessary in order to change the slope of their deterioration, with the goal that their eyes last until they die. (Kind of like treating glaucoma—but things can go bad fast if you make the wrong choice.)

> **Blue box break** for folks in developing countries, where patients are coming in with awful disease and awful control. These patients just need a ton of laser—often several thousand spots, especially if you have no access to vitrectomy and laser is your only option. You still have to try to break up such heavy treatment into a few sessions to avoid even more side effects, but there is no role for trying the gentler approaches outlined below. Good luck.

In fact, there is a wide assortment of treatments being essayed by retina specialists to try to minimize collateral damage from a PRP, ranging from undetectable micropulse treatment to minimal scatter techniques. The crucial thing is that if you do use a milder treatment, you and the patient have to understand that you are shackled together for eternity. You have to watch these patients and make sure they don't get little nubbins of neo around the areas of lighter treatment, and you have to be prepared to bite the bullet and fill in treatment as needed. You also want to have a good feel for which patients need heavy treatment— sometimes, treatment that is far denser than the DRS guidelines. It is very dangerous to fritter away time doing light treatments in such patients; you have to accept the risk of side effects to get aggressive proliferative disease under control quickly.

So keep the above contradictory koan in mind as you read the following on how to do a PRP...

Hey, here is a real Buddhist koan:

A monk asked Zhaozhou, "What is the meaning of the ancestral teacher's coming from the West?" Zhaozhou said, "The cypress tree in front of the hall."

Now how cool is that?

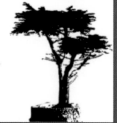

FIRST, A REVIEW OF SOME BASICS

Take care of any macular edema. You can really mess someone up if you put in an aggressive PRP when they have poorly controlled macular edema; the edema can get much worse. The best way to avoid this is to treat the edema and then start doing a gentle PRP (specific techniques to use are discussed below). If the patient has pre-proliferative disease or mild proliferative disease, you definitely have time to do all this slowly and carefully. It gets trickier if the edema is bad and the proliferative disease needs rapid treatment, too—you may have to simply treat the edema and start the PRP at the same time. Incidentally, if there is a lot of edema knocking the vision down, you might want to refer the patient out if you have the option of doing so—or at least call to get the latest thoughts about how to treat such a patient. Your friendly neighborhood retina specialist may want to proactively intervene with intravitreal therapy to protect the macula and allow safer, more effective treatment. See Chapter 11 for details.

The positioning and setup for doing the laser are similar to those discussed in Chapter 7, the chapter that is not really about doing a treatment for macular edema. Because a PRP tends to be much more intense than a macular laser, you really want to make sure the patient is comfortable and you *really* want to warn the patient about the increased discomfort that accompanies a PRP, especially if their only prior experience is with focal lasers.

Chapter 15 is specifically about controlling pain when doing a PRP, but it is worth discussing a few things right here, because you need to convey some of this to the patient from the start. It turns out that each spot you place—even if it is the exact same type of burn—can vary extremely in terms of discomfort. This is probably due to how close the spots are to the nerves in the suprachoroidal space. The greatest discomfort tends to occur in the mid-periphery, especially in the horizontal and diagonal clock hours where the nerves are more prominent. Although you usually cannot see the nerves themselves, you can often antici- pate increased pain when you move toward the vortex veins or more prominent choroidal veins—places where the nerves are more likely to be. This is really the case if there is extra pigment lying alongside the veins; this makes the burns hotter. Sometimes you can even detect the whiter coloration of a nerve, for instance in the horizontal meridians where the long ciliary nerves run. It makes sense to avoid these areas, or at least go lightly—both for pain control and to minimize effects on pupil function and accommodation. (See Chapter 16 on complications.)

However, even if you follow the above anatomic guidelines, you will find that many times you can be working in an area that is utterly unremarkable and suddenly the patient yelps in pain. You need to warn them in advance that this unexpected change in discomfort can happen. If they are not forewarned about this, and if you do hit a hot spot, they may think that you have cranked up the power and that you are trying to blow their head off—because that is what it can feel like. They can then get very skittish about the rest of the treatment because you hurt them in a way they were not prepared for. It is one thing to tell the patient that a procedure is uncomfortable, and it is another thing to have an unexpected burst of pain when neither you nor the patient expects it.

You should warn them about this and let them know that if it does happen, they should tell you. Then you can avoid the site of discomfort. Even if you warned them, however, it can be difficult to finish because once you hit a spot like this they can get nervous and their threshold of pain can change.

Also, be aware that some patients are exquisitely sensitive to this sudden change in pain, and may rapidly faint due to a vasovagal response. If you warn them about the possibility of both pain and fainting in advance, everyone pres- ent will be less frantic if the patient slowly melts down to the ground. If a pa- tient does tell you that they are starting to feel hot or light-headed, you should discontinue the laser immediately and order them to either lower their head between their legs or lie down on the floor. This is really important; once they start to go vasovagal, it may only be a matter of seconds before they convert the potential energy of their head into kinetic energy—a bad thing given all the sharp edges that are present in your lasering area. Sometimes it helps to put a cool washcloth on their forehead and you can even create a Victorian level of drama if you want to use smelling salts. (On the other hand, don't get cavalier and assume every light-headed patient is simply getting vasovagal. Remember that this group of patients may also be getting hypoglycemic or may even have a true emergency like a heart attack—make sure you monitor such a patient until they improve appropriately.)

GETTING STARTED

Having done all the talk to get the patient ready, it is now time to do the walk. First, you have to choose your weapon, or at least its color. At the beginning of the book it was assumed that you have a green laser, but it is worth noting that the other colors can come in handy when doing a PRP. No study has shown that any wavelength is superior in terms of the ultimate outcome, but just like it is nice to have different wrenches to work on a car, it is nice to know that different colors can be helpful in certain situations. Different wrenches don't cost $40,000, though, so don't feel like you have to run out and get another laser—this is simply an option to be aware of.

An example of a situation in which a different wavelength can be useful is when there are a lot of media opacities, such as a hemorrhage or a nuclear sclerotic cataract. In this case, you may want to use a redder wavelength because there is less scattering relative to green. An infrared laser can be even more effective at getting through such opacities, but it is trickier to use. (You should check the Appendix if you are going to use this wavelength.) Fortunately, you can get most routine jobs done with a green laser. If you really need to go to sky-high powers, though, you may want to refer the patient out to someone who has other wavelengths in order to avoid some of the complications discussed in upcoming chapters.

Next, remember that the spot size you set on the laser may end up being very different from what you get on the retina, especially if you are using a wide-field indirect lens. Refer to back Chapter 4 for the details—but the important thing is to know the magnification factor for the lens you are using. For instance, a very wide-field lens can double the spot size: If you are set at 500 microns on the slit lamp, you can end up placing 1,000-micron spots on the retina—and these are really huge, painful spots. (It is likely you would be using equally massive powers, and between the power and the pain, you would quickly realize your settings were unnecessarily harsh.) You should also remember that the number of spots you need to use is very dependent on the spot size. For instance, if you want to do a "standard" Diabetic Retinopathy Study PRP of 1,500 spots that are 500 microns in size—but you are using a smaller spot size—you can't just put in 1,500 spots and quit. You have to increase the number of spots you place so that you cover the same area that would have been covered by 500-micron burns (Figure 3).

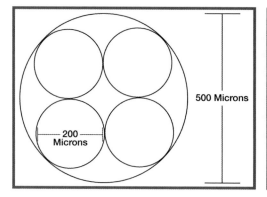

Figure 3. It takes at least four 200-micron spots to fill a 500-micron spot (the π-r-squared thing). If you want to place a certain "dose" of PRP based on the 500-micron burn size, then you have to increase the number of spots you place, depending on how many of your burns it takes to equal the area of a 500-micron spot.

500 Microns

200 Microns

How hot do you make the burns? It is hard to photograph the kind of burn that you actually see when you do a laser, because burns tend to soften rapidly after treatment—they also spread out a bit. The ETDRS asked for medium-white burns as seen in Figure 4, and this is fairly standard. Note the whitening in the center of most burns—if you are getting a much whiter burn, you are probably running too hot, and you should turn down the power.

Figure 5 shows a spread of different intensities. Many specialists feel that you can use lighter intensities (note, in the figure, the milder, grayish burns without any white center). One problem is that over time you will see that milder burns may not form scars as large as the original burn—so you can end up with less area treated than you had planned at the time of treatment. There are no long-term studies that prove you can get DRS results with burns that are less intense than the DRS standard, but in a patient with early, slowly progressive disease, it may be reasonable to use a lighter burn intensity and follow the patient closely to be sure their disease remains quiescent.

Figure 4 is also the standard density for a full PRP—the spots are about one-half burn width apart. The ETDRS had a "mild scatter" treatment arm, with fewer burns that were spaced further apart, and it is shown in Figure 6 for comparison. This milder pattern resulted in the middle (yellow) line in Figure 2. It is clearly not as effective as a full PRP, and most experts would not go this lightly—or at least not for the full treatment. Still, it gives you an idea of what has been tried and what to expect so you don't have to reinvent the wheel.

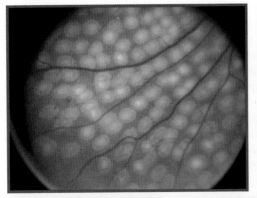

Figure 4. This is the ETDRS gold standard for burn intensity and density for a full scatter PRP. If you do less than this, you could get, uh, burned—but some patients may do quite well with less. Note that laser burns tend to spread out shortly after treatment, so the actual treatment density was a bit less than this. (Courtesy of the Early Treatment Diabetic Retinopathy Study Group)

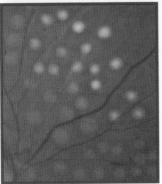

Figure 5. Variable-intensity burns with the upper burns being similar to ETDRS standards and the lower, grayer burns representing a milder approach. Note that you can see some of the choroidal detail through the lighter burns, but the whiteness of the heavier burns obscures the underlying choroid. This can help you decide how hot your burns are. Truth in advertising moment: This image was Photoshop'd to simulate the burns. It is hard to justify doing this to a patient for didactic reasons.

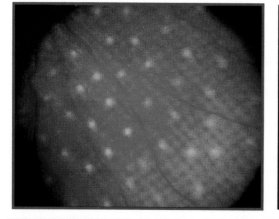

Figure 6. The ETDRS photo showing the pattern used for the "mild scatter" treatment arm. This is a very light pattern, but it may work in older patients with mild, slow disease. It is the pattern that resulted in the middle line in Figure 2—not as effective as a full scatter pattern, but it still had a treatment effect. (Courtesy of the Early Treatment Diabetic Retinopathy Study Group)

Incidentally, when this chapter suggests a given number of spots, it is assumed that these are equivalent to 500-micron spots. You will likely prefer to use smaller spots (for instance, for patient comfort), so you will need to adjust the actual number of spots you place, as outlined above. Also, when this chapter refers to a "standard DRS PRP" it means about 1,500 500-micron spots.

AMOUNT, STAGING, & FREQUENCY OF TREATMENT

There is a tendency to feel as though it is some sort of emergency when a patient presents with mild asymptomatic neovascularization. Do not surrender to the temptation to slag the retina simply because you see some vessels that look disturbing. Such vessels are unlikely to change over a few weeks, and most of the acute complications from PRP occur with aggressive treatment delivered all at once. In some ways, the situation is analogous to a patient who presents with long-standing severe hypertension: If you aggressively bring the blood pressure down far and fast you can give them a stroke, but if you gently work it down you can save them safely. It seems as though diabetic eyes function in a similar fashion. Eyes that present with early proliferative disease have been living in an ischemic milieu for quite some time. They can be rather fragile, and if you jump with 1,500 spots all at once, you are very likely to create permanent changes in the macula—as well as an extremely unhappy patient. As will be discussed below, it is often best to start slowly with a few hundred spots if you can.

Make no mistake; there are some situations in which time is not your friend. Patients with lots of very angry-looking vessels, very ischemic retinas and active hemorrhaging can go bad fast. The concern is that the extensive neovascularization evolves into dense fibrous tissue, causing severe traction that no amount of complex vitrectomy can undo. Wasting time doing a slow gentle PRP in such a patient can be disastrous. These patients are often younger Type 1 diabetics with a history of poor compliance, but any demographic can be affected. Such patients do need a lot of laser, even if it means risking side effects, because just about any laser complication is better than where the eye is heading. In this type of situation, you may want to bite the bullet and put in a thousand spots at first, and then repeat weekly until the patient is controlled or hemorrhages and needs surgery. In fact, if you have a patient who looks this bad and you are considering this type of treatment, you should strongly consider just referring them to a retina specialist. ASAP. This is not to strip you of your prerogatives as a Renaissance Comprehensive Ophthalmologist—but you should recognize that these patients can do abysmally, with even specialist care. There will be lots of bread-and-butter diabetics for you to treat who don't need subspecialty intervention, so consider sending these scary-bad patients off if you can. If you really, really want to treat such misery, you may need to find yourself a retina fellowship...

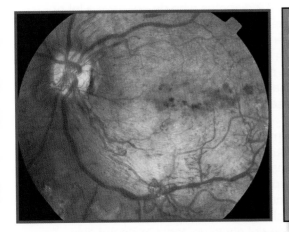

Figure 7. This is a very sick eye—most commonly seen in younger patients with a history of poor control. Note the swollen, beaded veins and all of the smaller intraretinal vessels that seem to start and stop in no clear pattern. Also, note the neovascularization—it is not large, but the vessels are thick and succulent in a way that bodes poorly for the patient. The blotchy hemorrhages in the macula suggest a lot of ischemia, and you are caught between the Scylla and Charybdis of doing a fast, aggressive PRP, yet trying not to blow out the fragile macula. Consider referring if you can—skillfully balancing all the treatment variables in this eye may be very important to the final outcome.

Also, are you waiting for a little chart on spot size, duration and power for a PRP? It would be nice to have a standard setting for all of your PRPs, but hopefully you are realizing that there are so many factors that using one setting for all PRPs is like telling Rembrandt that he could only use one paintbrush. With experience you will automatically come up with tailor-made settings for each patient based on a number of variables. These variables will include things such as how aggressively you want to treat the patient, their degree of pigmentation, the presence of media opacities, the location of the treatment and even your estimate of their pain threshold. All of these are discussed at various points in this chapter and throughout the book.

However, you do need to begin somewhere, so here are some basic numbers to try:

Most feel it is best to start with a duration of 0.1 second—this is a nice middling length of time that will not be too likely to let you get in trouble. A good starting spot size is around 350 to 500 microns at the retina (remember the effect of the contact lens on spot size). For the "average" patient, this duration and spot size usually means that you will want to start with a power of about 200 milliwatts and slowly increase it until you get burns similar to those seen in the photos. Don't hesitate to start at an even lower power if the media is crystal clear and/or there is a lot of pigment—you can always turn it up but you can't undo a spot that is too hot.

You can then gradually increase the power—say, by 20- to 50-milliwatt increments—until you start to see a slight graying of the retina. Once you begin to see a change it is likely that you only need to turn it up about 50 milliwatts more in order to get a standard burn. Another clue that you are getting close to the right power is that the patient will often tell you that they are beginning to feel it. You should probably not stray very much from settings like this until you are starting to get an intuitive feel for how the retina responds to your treatment, but once you have some experience you will find these settings way too restrictive.

How much do you treat?

This is the question. As the PRP koan implies, less is more—unless they go blind from your doing less. Then less was not enough, and you should have done more—unless they have problems from doing more, in which case you should have done less. You get the point. There are some guidelines, though, to help you decide where to start if you want to do something other than a "one size fits all" PRP.

There are some patients who seem to do well with smaller amounts of laser. These are generally older patients with Type 2 diabetes who do not have a lot of aggressive neovascularization. This is especially true if you are treating an older diabetic at an earlier stage, such as severe NPDR or low-risk PDR. As outlined above, if you decide to go conservative on your treatment, you are obligated to pay close attention to the patient, and the patient must understand that follow up is very important. If there is any sign that things are not responding appropriately, you will simply need to add more laser.

On the other hand, younger patients with more ischemic retinas and aggressive disease may require thousands and thousands of spots to just partially control the process. Accelerated medical problems can add to proliferative disease as well—a patient with renal failure or bad hypertension can kill off retinal vessels in a way that really powers up the neovascular stimulus. Finally, a patient with known poor control (or poor compliance) should get fairly heavy treatment to ensure stopping the disease even if they do not show up again or do not ever check their glucose levels.

For instance, a 70- to 80-year-old patient with Type 2 diabetes who is slowly developing PDR may only need 600 to 1,000 spots to slow things down enough until they exit the Grand Illusion. A 50-ish or 60-ish patient in a similar situation may need something closer to a standard PRP, especially if they have poor control or are progressing quickly. Thirties to forties may be fine with this same dose, but often need an extra "half of a PRP dose" for security (say, an extra 500 to 700 spots). Twenty-somethings are likely to be Type 1 patients who were poorly controlled—otherwise they would not get their disease so early. These patients may need two or three times a usual PRP dose, and often quickly.

NOTE: The above are just rough approximations. Each patient is different—gather some experience and use your judgment.

Is there a maximum number of spots? A study looking at this considered 6,500 500-micron spots to represent about the upper limit.[3] That is a lot of spots—maybe four to five times the amount of the standard DRS PRP—and other studies have gone even higher. The point is that you can put in a lot of laser and still stay away from the important bits of the retina. You can even use the 6,500 number to reassure patients about how much head room you have if they feel that you are destroying their eye with 1,500 hundred spots. Please forgive the repetition, but, if you think you need to keep putting in spots like this, you really should refer—with the intravitreal treatments and early vitrectomy it may be possible to spare patients this type of Total War ablation. (By the way, the maximum number of spots reported in the literature is 11,513 from back in the Eighties.[4] It is unlikely you will ever need to go there.)

Over how many sessions do you put in the treatment?

For the "average" patient with early PDR there is not a lot of time pressure, so it makes sense to start with gradual treatment applied over at least two, and usually three, sessions. Although the original studies often did all the treatment in one session—and it is within two standard deviations of accepted care to do it that way—such an approach can be asking for trouble. One-stop shopping with a PRP almost always requires retrobulbar anesthesia with the attendant risks. There is also a higher risk of problems such as angle-closure glaucoma and exudative choroidal or retinal detachments (see Chapter 16). Even two sessions can push it, especially in a fragile eye. Three sessions seems to work best with mild disease. There is less of a shock to the eye, and patients are more likely to tolerate the discomfort without needing a block.

> **Another factor** that can be very important in deciding how to treat a patient is whether you think they will be compliant. Although a wayward patient is not the ideal patient for risking side effects from aggressive treatment, it may be better to treat such patients quickly over fewer sessions before they wander off and stop seeing anyone. It can be very gratifying to see such patients years later and find that they can still see and function in society thanks to the fact that you put in enough laser before they disappeared (even if they are still bitching about how they hated the laser).

Here is an example of why one should start slowly if possible: Doing a PRP always carries some risk of worsening macular edema, and it seems the more you do at one setting, the greater the risk. In fact, there are some patients who may be unbelievably sensitive to this effect. These patients don't turn up very often, but you will certainly know if you stumble across one. Such patients may go from 20/20 to 20/50 for weeks with as few as 200 or 300 gentle laser spots. If you happen to hit one of these patients very hard with the first treatment, you can knock them down to count-fingers and they may never completely recover. And it can happen even if you dutifully treated their edema prior to doing any PRP.

Fortunately, this type of severe decreased vision after a PRP is unusual, but it still makes sense to go slowly with every patient with milder disease. You may want to initiate panretinal photocoagulation with as little as 200 to 400 spots— sometimes even less if you are really worried—and then plan on adding the full amount over one to two additional sessions, depending upon how the patient tolerates the first treatment. This will usually keep you out of permanent trouble if you come across a patient who is very sensitive to PRP. If you do have a patient whose vision drops, you should wait to let things return to baseline before adding more treatment (if the proliferative disease will let you). Sometimes these patients even need to be treated in small doses over six to eight sessions. (Such patients may get a bit frustrated over this experience, so consider a second opinion to keep everyone happy.) Another option in patients like this is intravitreal therapy to keep the macula dry while the PRP is being placed.[5] The important point is to be flexible and never approach the number of sessions with that "one size fits all" mentality.

> **This blue box likely applies only to docs practicing in America.**
>
> Chapter 21 discusses in detail the socioeconomic issues involved in treating diabetics, but there is one issue that needs to be covered right here. Most insurance companies will pay for a PRP only once every 90 days. The thinking is that they only have to pay once, and that payment will cover as many treatments as are needed for the three-month period. You don't have to have a Nobel Prize in economics to realize that there is, therefore, a strong urge to do every PRP in one session — or as few sessions as possible — in order to maximize revenue per unit of time in the clinic.
>
> Please, please, please ignore this urge. If you are in the early phases of your training, you are likely untainted and this admonition will seem ridiculous. If you have a practice and a family to pay for, you may notice that a sense of frustration can slowly creep into your soul as you circle the "no charge" line on a bunch of lasers. Recognize that the PRP reimbursement is structured so that these extra visits are taken into account — you are in fact being paid to do several treatments. Consider only what is best for the patient, and pinch yourself strongly if you find that you are even remotely thinking about this as you plan a given patient's treatment.
>
> (As an aside within an aside, you may run across patients treated in the really old days when PRPs were paid for visit by visit. Having a patient tell you that they were brought back 12 times over six months to get a little bit of PRP each time will help you understand that maybe the present payment system isn't so bad.)

You also have to be flexible about how often you schedule each session; patients with aggressive PDR may need treatment every week, but treating patients every two weeks is probably best. It has been shown using OCT that even a healthy macula will swell a bit after a PRP. If patients are treated every week, it takes longer for their maculae to recover from this swelling than if the PRP sessions are spread out every two weeks.[6] (And patients in this particular study started with relatively healthy maculae.*) It seems safe to assume that if a patient has a compromised macula, it may be risky to do PRPs spaced a week apart — best to spread things out a bit if the proliferative disease will let you.

Another reason to go with every-two-week treatment is that it is often hard to see where you treated if you bring them back after a week — it often takes about two weeks for the spots to become more visible from scarring. (Finesse point: You can usually identify previous spots — even if you can't see them clinically — in the backscatter of your laser light as described in Chapter 8.)

However, issues beyond what is best for the eye can sometimes play a role in deciding how many sessions to do and how far apart they should be spaced. Some patients may risk losing their job if they are absent too often, so be sensitive to such needs and adjust the treatment plan accordingly. (If the retinopathy is mild, you might be able to treat at longer intervals so there is more time between days off for the patient — this is better than risking macular problems by

---

* One does not get to use a nifty word like maculae very often, yet here it occurs twice in one paragraph. Excellent.

stuffing a lot of laser into one session just to make their boss happy.)

What if they need bilateral treatment? It is always a bit dicey to do bilateral PRPs right off the bat. If you have one of those patients with really fussy maculae, you can shut down their ability to function for quite a while if you treat both eyes at once. Even if you want to get treatment started quickly in both eyes, it usually makes sense to treat one eye first so you and the patient can see how the eye responds. You can start treating the fellow eye in a few days and adjust your approach depending on how the first eye behaves. If things go well, and the patient doesn't mind having both eyes blurry at the same time, then you can treat bilaterally to save visits. If things don't go well, then you will likely need to alternate eyes at each treatment. This can turn into a lot of visits, but so be it if it makes the treatment safer.

What if they have a hemorrhage when they present?

First of all, remember the caveats in Chapter 12—make sure that you are dealing with proliferative disease and not another cause, such as a retinal tear. If the patient does have proliferative disease, then the treatment protocol depends on the amount of blood present. If there is a dense hemorrhage with no view—and they have no history of prior laser—you should refer for early vitrectomy to clear the blood out and get in laser before permanent damage occurs.

If there is a dense hemorrhage but you can see some retina, you should treat as much as you can (assuming you can be sure the posterior retina is safe with a B scan). The goal of the faster treatment is to get laser in before further hemorrhage obscures your ability to treat the eye. If you can get in enough laser, you may be able to stabilize the eye and give it a chance to clear without the need for vitrectomy. If there is not a lot of room, you might want to just treat all the retina you can see at the first session. This is especially true if there are areas of loculated hemorrhage being held in place by the cortical vitreous. These loculations can rupture and if the blood spreads throughout the central vitreous you will lose your ability to treat previously visible portions of the retina.

If there is more room, you may want to be a bit more conservative in order to avoid complications related to an excessive PRP; perhaps treat in two sessions a week apart using a fairly large number of spots (say 500 to 1,000 to treat the inferior retina, followed by enough to fill in the remaining fundus at the next session). This is more aggressive than usual, but not enough to pulverize the eye. Whether you treat all at once or in divided doses, recognize that there really is no incorrect approach as long as you are thinking about what you are doing. (By the way, patients with a vitreous hemorrhage are often best treated first with a wide-field indirect lens to slip around the blood as much as possible, then with a Goldmann three mirror for squeaking treatment out to the far periphery. You will often have a clear view of the far anterior retina because the blood can't get through the vitreous base.)

If the hemorrhage is mild and the patient has good vision, you should consider going slower if the proliferative disease is not very aggressive-looking. There is often more time than you would expect between hemorrhages in eyes with mild disease, and you are unlikely to "miss an opportunity" by dividing the treatments in patients who are less sanguineous. Although the presence of the blood is often as scary to you as it is to the patient, consider restraining yourself in order to avoid damaging the macula. (If you are going to treat over multiple sessions, it does make sense to tell such patients to give you a call if they think the hemorrahge is getting worse—you can bring them in and finish the treatment quickly if necessary.)

Also, remember that if you are treating a diabetic with a mild hemorrhage, you have to remind them that you can only indirectly control their "bad blood vessels" with the laser. They need to know that the blood may get much worse, depending on the capricious nature of their disease. You especially need to remind them that the laser will not make the blood in their vision disappear overnight. Don't be surprised if you have to repeat this last point if you call the patient to see how they are doing after the laser. Patients have a strong tendency to assume that the laser will immediately solve a problem that the diabetes has been working for years to create.

> **It turns out** that patients with hemorrhages may end up being some of your most grateful patients if the hemorrhage clears after the laser (and it usually does if the disease is relatively mild). They will understand exactly where they were headed, and even if it takes a few months for the blood to wash out, they will greatly appreciate the fact that you saved them with your laser skills. It makes one wish that every diabetic would just have a little teeny hemorrhage as soon as they start to get some neovascularization. Then they would understand why we do this...

Where should you treat?

The standard DRS protocol called for non-specifically treating from the posterior pole to the equator, but, as with corneas, custom ablation is often the way to go.

For the "standard" treatment, the posterior border usually starts a disc width from the nerve and just outside the major arcades around the macula. The temporal treatment line is usually two to four disc diameters temporal to the fovea (Figure 8). Treatment is then carried out to the point where your contact lens can't easily see through the patient's lens—usually to an area anterior to the equator.

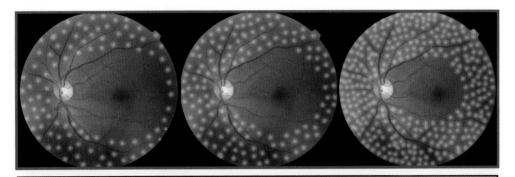

Figure 8. A triptych of approaches to choosing the posterior border to a PRP. These are also Photoshop'd—one would be reluctant to put in this much laser all around the posterior pole at one treatment unless absolutely necessary. The middle would be about standard; the one on the left would be very light (i.e., an elderly patient with mild disease), and the right would be a very aggressive treatment for refractory disease.

The actual borders that you choose depend on how severe the disease is. There is a common clinical impression that "one spot in the back is equal to two or more on the side," probably because the posterior retina is so much thicker and there are a lot more cells to generate vasoproliferative factors. Bad disease may, therefore, need treatment that extends further into the posterior pole. For instance, some patients need treatment using smaller spots just inside the arcades and two disc diameters temporal to the fovea. Sometimes the treatment needs to be even closer to the fovea (for instance, if the angiogram shows that there is a lot of ischemia temporal to the fovea driving the neovascularization). You can also get a bit closer to the nerve, but most folks stay at least 500 microns away to avoid thermal damage to the disc. However, moving into areas this close to the center with panretinal photocoagulation is not without risk. If you find that you are considering this, you may want to refer the patient to a retina specialist because the patient may benefit from anti-VEGF treatment and/ or vitrectomy to gain control and perhaps avoid the need to ablate retina so close to the center of vision.

> **It is helpful to** use an angiogram with views of the periphery to guide your treatment. The FA will delineate the areas of capillary dropout nicely (especially the newer wide-field angiography techniques, as shown in Figure 1 in Chapter 12). This allows very targeted treatment. There is, as yet, no study proving that such an approach is better, but it does seem more intuitively satisfying, and photos of the border between dying and normal retina are great visual aids to help patients understand the problem.

In patients with less aggressive disease, it is possible to stay farther away from the posterior pole. For instance, Blankenship did a study on the effect of bringing treatment just inside the arcades, versus bringing treatment only to within two or three disc diameters of the arcades (Figure 9).[7] Both groups did well, and there were fewer patients with macular problems in the peripheral group. However, the follow up was only six months in this study and patients usually have decades over which they can generate vasoproliferative substances from lightly treated retina. Nevertheless, this is one approach to consider in a patient who needs a lot of PRP but also has a lot of macular edema; more peripheral treatment can start to get things under control with less risk of worsening the macular edema. The patient will need to be watched, and it is likely you will need to fill in closer to the center, but hopefully by then the macula will be more stable and the treatment can be done more safely.

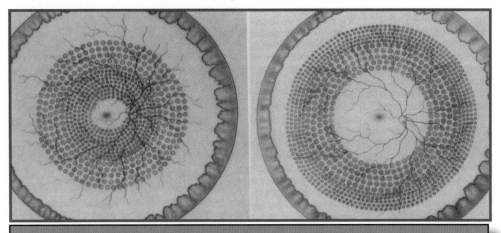

Figure 9. Patterns used in a study comparing central versus peripheral PRP. Over six months, the results were similar and the peripheral group had less macular edema. (Blankenship GW, A clinical comparison of central and peripheral argon laser panretinal photocoagulation for proliferative diabetic retinopathy. Ophthalmology 95:170-7, 1988. Copyright Elsevier)

The temporal area can be problematic, because aggressive treatment in this location seems to be associated with the worsening of any macular edema. However, this area also tends to have a lot of thick ischemic retina, which can cause trouble if not treated aggressively. In general, there is a tendency for non-retina specialists to be too conservative in treating temporally, and because this area can develop neovascularization years down the road, it should be watched closely if it is not treated. One sign that trouble is developing is if the untreated region "re-acquires" findings associated with severe NPDR. In other words, if an area starts to have increasing intraretinal hemorrhages with IRMA and venous beading (as in the 4-2-1 rule) it is likely that area needs additional PRP. An angiogram can again be helpful for guiding treatment, because it will clearly show any ischemia. You don't want to cream this area all at once if you can help it, but don't hesitate to move in if you are not happy with more conservative results.

Another subtlety of panretinal photocoagulation is to use variable spot density in different areas of the fundus. For instance, it seems reasonable to use a lower density of spots superiorly and nasally if the patient does not have severe disease. These areas correlate to the inferior and temporal visual field, which are the most useful portions, particularly in older patients who may have trouble ambulating. You can then treat the inferior retina more confluently (changes in the superior visual field tend to be less noticeable—unless your patient is a fighter pilot or spelunker). You can also treat more confluently in the temporal retina, which is generally compensated for by the nasal retina in the fellow eye.

Getting Way Out There

Most of the time you do not need to go out as far as possible with a PRP; a bit anterior to the equator will do. On occasion you may want to treat everything, for instance in a very ischemic eye or if there is a hemorrhage that prevents treatment of the usual sites. You may also have a patient who is blocked or not very cooperative, which can make it hard to even get to the equator, let alone get to the ora. You have some options:

1. Use all the lenses at your disposal—generally a Goldmann can go out the farthest in a phakic patient and a wide-field indirect contact lens can go out the farthest in a pseudophakic patient.
2. Delivering laser through a binocular indirect ophthalmoscope is a great technique, but is usually not available to a comprehensive ophthalmologist. If this is an option, see the suggested reading section at the end of this chapter for a good reference on this approach.
3. Have the patient look in the direction you are treating or, if they are blocked or uncooperative, torque the eye with the lens, as discussed in Chapter 4.
4. If the eye is blocked, you or someone you trust can push in on the eye to indent the periphery and bring it into view. This often requires three hands, and you can get a very hot burn if you treat right on the hump that is created, so be careful.
5. There is an obscure device known as an Eisner Cone that fits behind the eyelids and provides a way to indent the periphery when using a Goldmann-type lens. This is not easy to use, and it is hard to find, but it is good to be aware of. You would probably be better off getting an indirect ophthalmoscope attachment for your laser if you really want to get this advanced.
6. There is one final move that can be very helpful, and that involves coordinating the position of the patient's head and the angle of your slit lamp. Sometimes, if you have them turn to the side a bit and you swing your slit lamp in the other direction, you can get a few extra degrees of visualization in the periphery. You can also raise and lower the laser table to get a little better view of the superior and inferior retina, respectively, as the patient's head tilts up and down at the slit lamp.

These techniques don't always work but sometimes they come in handy for diabetics or patients that have retinal tears in the periphery. YMMV.

The DRS called for the direct, confluent treatment of flat patches of neovascularization in the periphery in order to stamp them out. It is not clear whether this is really necessary, because small patches of flat NVE tend to be benign, anyway, and an effective PRP pattern will automatically take care of them. If you feel you have to treat directly, though, do be careful, because very aggressive laser will thin out the retina. If traction then develops, these atrophic areas can tear and allow the retina to detach. Most specialists no longer do this.

Although one may or may not want to treat small patches of flat neovascularization, there is agreement that one should go lightly in areas of pronounced gliosis and extensive neovascularization. These areas will very likely contract with time, and it is important to avoid treating them with heavy confluent burns due to the risk of stimulating aggressive contraction and the risk of eventual hole formation. If traction already exists, or if the retina appears excessively thin, you definitely want to avoid creating a hot spot, because if you poke a hole in one of these taut areas both you and the patient will be sorry very quickly. Repairing combined traction/rhegmatogenous detachments in diabetics is not easy, and the visual results are usually not impressive, even if the surgery is successful. If a hole forms the vitreoretinal surgeon has to religiously strip off anything that can cause traction—something that is very tricky in areas of retina that are already atrophic. Just be careful when treating around places like this.

Where to stage the treatment

Most people will treat the inferior fundus at the first session. Treatment in this area tends to cause fewer symptoms because the inferior fundus corresponds to less useful visual field. Treating this area first also ensures that it is treated in the event that a hemorrhage occurs; the blood tends to settle inferiorly and preclude further treatment. Subsequent treatments will then fill in nasally, superiorly and temporally. Because there is a sense that treating temporal to the fovea is most likely to exacerbate macular edema, it is a good idea to close the temporal loop in at least two steps.

Figure 10 shows how you might treat over two or three sessions. The three-session approach is probably the safest for patients who have early disease and for whom there is no time pressure.

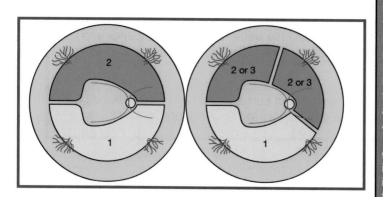

Figure 10. Suggested two- and three-stage PRP patterns. (Reproduced, with permission, from Folk JC, Pulido JS, Ophthalmology Monographs 11: Laser Photocoagulation of the Retina and Choroid, American Academy of Ophthalmology, 1997.) By the way, this is a great book for laser treatment in general—lots of timeless info about lasering many different diseases.

One of the more difficult things about treating proliferative disease is that, as a conscientious physician, you may find yourself empathizing with your patient in terms of their absolute hatred of panretinal photocoagulation. It can be especially rough if they want to forego retrobulbar anesthesia for whatever reason—you can end up feeling every spot with them. All of this can make you want to try to "help them" by doing the least amount of PRP possible, and it can be easy to grossly undertreat patients by doing this.

Unfortunately, treating proliferative retinopathy usually means you have to be cruel to be kind, and unless you are absolutely convinced that the proliferative disease is mild, you need to harden your heart a bit and put in the appropriate treatment. The next chapter will discuss all sorts of strategies to minimize the patient's discomfort and make the process easier, so you can get the right amount of treatment in with the least amount of pain for both of you.

(If this blue box makes no sense to you, please check the level of your empathy tank before it is too late.)

References and Suggested Reading

1.   Kaufman SC, Ferris FL, 3rd, Seigel DG, Davis MD, DeMets DL. Factors associated with visual outcome after photocoagulation for diabetic retinopathy. Diabetic Retinopathy Study Report #13. Invest Ophthalmol Vis Sci 1989;30:23-8.
2.   Early photocoagulation for diabetic retinopathy. ETDRS report number 9. Early Treatment Diabetic Retinopathy Study Research Group. Ophthalmology 1991;98:766-85.
3.   Reddy VM, Zamora RL, Olk RJ. Quantitation of retinal ablation in proliferative diabetic retinopathy. Am J Ophthalmol 1995;119:760-6.
4.   Aylward GW, Pearson RV, Jagger JD, Hamilton AM. Extensive argon laser photocoagulation in the treatment of proliferative diabetic retinopathy. Br J Ophthalmol 1989;73:197-201.
5.   Margolis R, Singh RP, Bhatnagar P, Kaiser PK. Intravitreal triamcinolone as adjunctive treatment to laser panretinal photocoagulation for concomitant proliferative diabetic retinopathy and clinically significant macular oedema. Acta Ophthalmol 2008;86:105-10.
6.   Shimura M, Yasuda K, Nakazawa T, Kano T, Ohta S, Tamai M. Quantifying alterations of macular thickness before and after panretinal photocoagulation in patients with severe diabetic retinopathy and good vision. Ophthalmology 2003;110:2386-94.
7.   Blankenship GW. A clinical comparison of central and peripheral argon laser panretinal photocoagulation for proliferative diabetic retinopathy. Ophthalmology 1988;95:170-7.

Friberg TR. Laser photocoagulation using binocular indirect ophthalmoscope laser delivery systems. Ophthalmic Surg Lasers 1995;26:549-59.

Folk JC, Pulido JS. Laser photocoagulation of the retina and choroid. San Francisco: American Academy of Ophthalmology, 1997.

Fong DS, Ferris FL. Practical Management of Diabetic Retinopathy. American Academy of Ophthalmology Focal Points 2003;21.

Davis MD, Blodi BA. Proliferative Diabetic Retinopathy. In: Ryan SJ. Retina, 4th ed. Philadelphia: Elsevier Mosby, 2006:v.2, pp 1285-1322.

Neubauer AS, Ulbig MW. Laser treatment in diabetic retinopathy. Ophthalmologica 2007;221:95-102.

Bloom, SM, Brucker, AJ. Laser Surgery of the Posterior Segment. Philadelphia: Lippincott Williams & Wilkins, 1997.

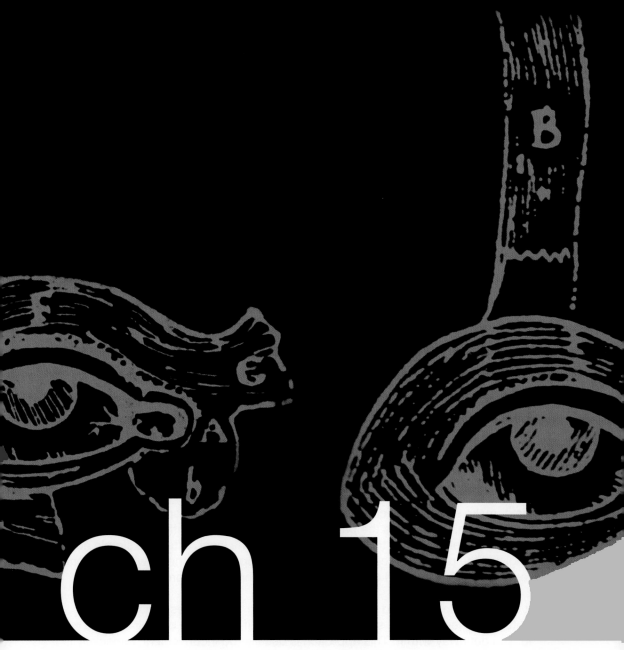

COITER *1572 erstmals beschrieben h*

ch 15

Doc, at Least It's Not as Bad as Having a Baby: Pain Control for PRPs.

Pain control can be a real problem, especially on a busy clinic day, when all you want to do is cook some retina and move on. It is a good idea to slow down and deal with this thoroughly, though, for three reasons:

1. It is a nice thing to do.
2. It is easier to get patients to return for follow up if the experience is not awful.
3. When patients sit around waiting for their endocrinology appointment, they will compare your treatment to the treatment that the other diabetics get. They will dump you if they find out that someone else makes the experience more pleasant than, say, the average Inquisition.

It may well be that as new laser technologies and new laser techniques are brought online, the whole issue of pain control will become much less of a problem. For instance, if gentler techniques such as the micropulse laser mentioned in Chapter 3 are proven to be effective in treating proliferative disease, then perioperative pain will be minimal. New delivery systems that can automatically apply multiple burns in rapid succession may also be helpful. However, new technology tends to be very expensive, and techniques that try to get by with less treatment than traditional ETDRS and DRS protocols are still investigational. As a result, this chapter will assume that you are doing traditional treatment with traditional tools.

There are a number of variables you can manipulate to make things more comfortable. The first is just to do what was mentioned in Chapter 7: Try to mentally put yourself in the patient's position, and try to anticipate what will scare them or make them uncomfortable. Always inform them about what you are about to do, and try to keep up a calm, soothing chatter while you are doing it—in other words, be a junior hypnotist.

Next, make sure the topical anesthesia has not worn off—especially during a long session. Sometimes the patient can't distinguish the difference between surface discomfort from the lens and pain from the laser. Often the simple act of giving the patient a break as you add more topical anesthesia will help them reset their pain threshold and allow you to get through the procedure.

It can also help to spread the treatment out over multiple sessions, perhaps putting in a few hundred spots at each session if the nature of their disease will let you get away with it. This approach is usually too inconvenient, especially if patients or family members have to take time off of work for each treatment, but this can work well for some patients as long as the proliferative disease is not progressing.

Some doctors feel that systemic medications will help. You can try anxiolytics or pain medicine by whatever route you feel comfortable. However, when you start tickling the long ciliary nerves it seems as though no amount of systemic medication can help. Nevertheless, remember that you have the option of using systemic treatment, and you will find an occasional anxious patient who does much better with a hit of Xanax while they are dilating.

There are also some variables on the laser you can play with. The two simplest things are to decrease the spot size and decrease the duration. Some lasers can go down to 0.02 seconds on the duration; this seems to help decrease the discomfort.[1] Remember the warnings in the chapter on laser wrangling, though. When you decrease the duration, you will have to compensate by turning up the power. This, in turn, means that there is less time for the heat to spread out in the tissues, and you may be more likely to get a hot burn if you are not paying very close attention to what you are doing—especially if you are also using a small spot and there is a lot of pigment variation in the fundus. You may want to get comfortable with longer durations first, and once you have a more intuitive sense of how the retina responds to your laser you can try going to these much shorter durations.

Also, as mentioned in the previous chapter, you will notice that patients will sometimes complain of a great deal of pain in one location of the fundus and have less pain in another. Most of the time you can correlate this with the location of the various ciliary nerves; for instance, pain is especially common near pigmented areas between the tributaries of vortex veins. Sometimes the phenomenon is random, and the patient will jump as you are treating a nondescript area of the fundus. You can always treat the less painful areas first and save the more painful ones for fill-in treatment, if necessary.

> **By the way**, there is a situation in which the technique in the previous paragraph can burn you, as well as the patient. If, in follow up, you are seeing a patient who has an odd, patchy PRP pattern, you can bet that the previous treating physician did this very thing as the laser was being placed. If you need to do a PRP fill on such a patient, it is guaranteed that every single one of your spots will be quite painful, no matter how you tweak the settings—and the patient will be convinced that you are a monster and their previous doctor was a saint. It always helps to warn patients that subsequent lasers can be more painful so they understand what is going on.

Another technique is to slow down the rate of fire. Sometimes, rapid laser treatment results in temporal summation and can make the experience more miserable. Slowing down the treatment a lot, however, can make the laser really drag on and on, and it may be better to move on to some sort of anesthetic injection if both you and the patient are getting frustrated by the long process.

If you do need to do regional anesthesia, the standard approach tends to be either a retrobulbar or peribulbar injection, depending on your preference. There is a general sense that a retrobulbar injection is more effective and faster, whereas a peribulbar technique may be safer (although it takes longer to work, and may require multiple injections, which can obviate any advantages). A full discussion is well beyond the scope of this book—in short, do what works best for you based on your experience.

> **In addition to full-blown orbital anesthesia,** you can occasionally get by with more localized injections. For instance, after numbing the conjunctiva with a pledget, you can place subconjunctival anesthesia, which will do a fairly good job of numbing the anterior portion of a quadrant of the fundus. Another option is to try a sub-Tenon's approach. Although a sub-Tenon's injection is unlikely to give you complete anesthesia of the globe, it can be very effective for treating a larger quadrant of the fundus, and may be safer than a retrobulbar injection. These are not techniques you are likely to use often, but they are good things to keep in your toolbox.

Of course, you need to clearly state the risks of performing local anesthesia, such as globe perforation, retrobulbar hemorrhage and even diplopia from inadvertent muscle injection. All of these things are unlikely, but if you treat a lot of diabetics, you will do a lot of retrobulbar injections, and the odds will tend to catch up with you at some point. You do not want such a complication to come as a surprise to the patient. Usually, however, if the patient is miserable from the laser they will be more than willing to accept the small risk of a numbing shot.

Oh, and don't forget to find out if the patient is on Coumadin. If they are, you may want to check an INR to make sure things are not too out-of-control prior to an injection (more on this in Chapter 25). It is very easy to forget to do this when things are busy, but a busy day is exactly when the retina gods will make you try to remember how to decompress an orbital hemorrhage in an anticoagulated patient...

> **Hey, sorry** to throw in two text boxes that are only two paragraphs apart, but it is worth pointing out that if a patient has a really high INR, yet you still need to get some laser in fast (i.e., neovascular glaucoma), it is a great time to use the less invasive anesthesia techniques mentioned in the preceding blue box.

Also, remember that people who have had Lasik or cataract surgery may now be refractively emmetropic, when in fact they still have big, pear-shaped eyes. Do not assume that an aggressive placement of your retrobulbar needle is safe just because patients are not wearing thick myopic spectacles. A needle through the retina tends to be worse than any degree of proliferative disease. Duh.

Finally, you should also have appropriate resuscitation equipment available, and your staff should check on patients shortly after performing an anesthetic injection in the office. Remember that if your anesthetic gets into the brain pan you do not want the patient to be alone when they stop breathing. Be especially alert for any patient who starts to complain of trouble swallowing or breathing within a few minutes of the injection—watch them carefully, and do not assume that they are just having a vasovagal response. Interesting factoid: There has been at least one case reported wherein a patient developed respiratory arrest from a retrobulbar, and when the patient recovered, he said that he was awake the whole time—he just could not talk or move during the episode.[2] Watch your language!

Whatever method you use to make your patients comfortable, your most useful tool is your clinical experience. It will not take long for you to realize that some patients do extremely well and other patients are likely to have real problems with the laser—and you will get a sense about which category a patient is in just by interacting with them well before you sit them down in the laser suite. (Insert, once again, the standard stereotype about the burly, tattooed male being unable to tolerate much of anything).

> **You will likely** find that a patient's ability to tolerate the laser decreases as you put in the treatments. Many patients can do well with the first two treatments, but end up needing an injection with the third. Just be flexible.

Also, recognize that some patients are unable to decide between the risk of an injection and the pain of the laser. Although modern medicine emphasizes informing patients and "letting them decide for themselves," this is a situation in which you may want to gently suggest that they try an injection one time to see how they like it. They will usually choose to use an injection henceforth, once they see how easy it is, and you will have avoided a very, very long session at the laser. (Understand that this is not a situation in which saving the doctor's time is more important than the patient's safety. Instead, what you are avoiding is a long, tedious session wherein both the doctor and the patient can become toxic. This is bad for everyone, and can lead to an unhappy patient who does not return for follow up, which is the worst outcome. In this case, the overall karma allows you to revert to being a typical movie doctor from 1948 and just telling the patient what to do—not a good idea in general, but very effective when used sparingly.)

Some doctors will routinely give retrobulbar injections to everyone because they make treatment faster. Although this does rev up the assembly line, the sheer number of injections inevitably increases the risk of a bad complication. Also, you will find that patients who have been in such a practice are often very grateful if they end up going to a doc who gives them a choice, rather than automatically giving them a retrobulbar. It is much better to take a little more time to sit the patient down and let them see what a PRP is like. This way, you can explain in advance the potential risks of regional anesthesia, and they can decide for themselves if they want to bail out and get a numbing shot. You will find that many patients can tolerate a fairly stiff dose of laser without automatic injections—it takes a little more time, but most patients appreciate being given the chance to decide (preceding paragraph notwithstanding!).

What about post-op pain?

Most of the bad pain tends to occur right at the time of the laser, and then resolves once the treatment is over. However, sometimes the pain shows up later and can be quite severe, especially if the patient was blocked and you put in a lot of treatment. First of all, you do need to see the patient if there is increasing pain. As will be discussed in the next chapter, you need to make sure the cornea, and, in particular, the intraocular pressure are OK because these things can cause pain that needs to be treated with something other than "take two aspirin and call me in the morning."

Most of the time the eye itself will be doing well, but the person attached to the eye will be miserable. If you do a lot of laser at one session, you may want to give them a topical steroid and cycloplegics to head this off. You can also try oral pain medicine, although many diabetics are not allowed to have nonsteroidals due to possible effects on kidney function. Diabetics can also get violently nauseated from narcotics due to GI motility problems combined with the tendency of eye pain to produce nausea. Sometimes simple things like a cool or warm compress can help, and on rare occasion the most merciful thing to do is to re-block the patient using a long-acting anesthetic. Usually, time is your best friend.

Some patients can even get so sick they throw themselves into diabetic ketoacidosis, so have a low threshold of referral to their internist, or even the emergency room, if they are telling you that they are having trouble keeping their food down or controlling their sugar. This type of severe problem seems more likely in younger patients with brittle disease.

In any event, if you do run into problems with post-op pain, be sure to note it in the chart; such patients benefit from doing the laser in smaller increments over longer intervals if at all possible.

References and Suggested Reading

1.   Al-Hussainy S, Dodson PM, Gibson JM. Pain response and follow-up of patients undergoing panretinal laser photocoagulation with reduced exposure times. Eye 2008;22:96-9.

2.   Simon MA, Cosgrove G, Zwillich CW, Chan ED. Respiratory arrest in the eye clinic. Chest 2001;119:1953-5.

Folk JC, Pulido JS. Laser photocoagulation of the retina and choroid. San Francisco: American Academy of Ophthalmology, 1997.

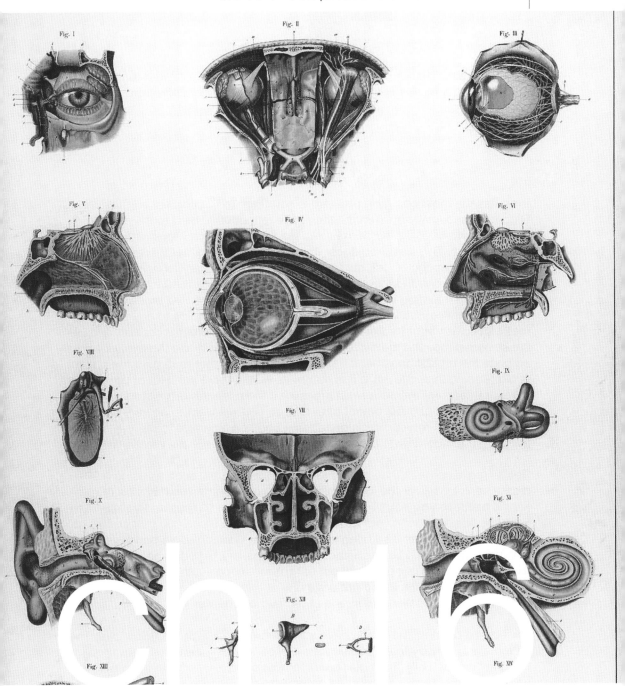

You Should Not Do Magic You Do Not Understand:
Complications of Laser Treatment

Although each chapter covers some of the complications related to treating diabetic retinopathy, it is probably a good idea to gather all the potential complications together in one place so you can be reminded why you spent years learning how to do this.

ANTERIOR SEGMENT COMPLICATIONS

Probably the most common problem is scruffing up the corneal epithelium. Diabetics, especially by the time they have retinopathy, tend to have a bad combination of decreased corneal sensation and anterior basement membrane abnormalities. This can predispose them to punctate epithelial erosions or even full-thickness epithelial defects from the use of the contact lens. Fortunately, this is not very common, and if there are symptoms they tend to be mild and self-limited—meaning that they are a perfect indication for all those artificial tear samples that keep building up in your cabinets. It also helps to rinse out the methylcellulose after treatment, both to increase the patient's comfort and because sometimes the methylcellulose can thicken and make the eye very irritated once the topical anesthetic has worn off. Don't forget to remind the patient to avoid rubbing their eye while it is numb, as well. If there are a lot of pre-existing anterior basement membrane changes, or if the patient has a history of getting a full thickness epithelial defect after a laser, you will want to be very careful with their epithelium. You can consider adding copious ointment to the eye or even patching it temporarily to protect the epithelium while the anesthetic wears off.

Really fragile corneas may need "no touch" techniques, such as using a 90-diopter lens to deliver the laser without using a contact lens. It is a bit of a hassle because you don't have as much control over the eye and you have to keep the lids open with your other fingers, but it is a technique that comes in handy at times. It has also been suggested that you can use a bandage contact lens underneath your laser contact lens if necessary.[2] Another option would be to deliver the laser using an indirect ophthalmoscope—although most general ophthalmologist's offices do not have one of these. If you are interested in doing this, there is an excellent reference at the end of Chapter 14.

Occasional patients may even have surface problems with the fellow eye. These patients are so busy trying to keep their fellow eye open and to fixate properly that they can actually dry it out, creating a lot of post-laser pain in an eye you never touched. Always encourage patients to periodically close their fixating eye, so as not to run into this problem. (By the way, this is particularly likely if you are treating both eyes at the same session. If they keep the eye you first treated wide open while you treat the second eye, they can really dry out the cornea because they are numb—especially if any methylcellulose is holding the anesthetic on the epithelium. You definitely need to remind them to close their first eye in this situation.)

It is also possible to cause corneal or lens burns with the laser, especially if you are using high powers. As mentioned in the chapter on contact lenses, the wide-field indirect lenses can actually result in high irradiance at the plane of the cornea or lens, especially with very large spot sizes. This becomes important if there are any opacities that might take up the laser on its way to the retina— such as eyelashes or bits of mascara stuck under the contact lens, or corneal pigmentation near the limbus.

A problem that was more common in the past was the occurrence of burns in the lens. This would happen if there was significant nuclear sclerosis: The yellowed lens would take up the laser (especially the blue-green wavelength that was more common back then). Patients would end up with very characteristic lenticular burns (see Figure 1).

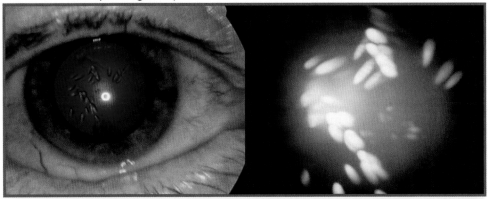

Figure 1. Lens burns seen with the red reflex and up close with direct illumination. With conservative powers and spot sizes, you will likely never see this, but be careful if you are using an indirect contact lens with large powers and spot sizes of 500 microns or more.

Other anterior segment complications include iatrogenic Aide's pupil, which can result from very heavy laser, especially anterior to the equator where the short ciliary nerves branch out to reach the ciliary body and iris. This probably will not have any significant visual consequences, but patients may get very fussy if they feel you have changed their appearance—not everyone wants to look like David Bowie. Basically, try not to use deep and heavy burns unless absolutely necessary, when treating over the long ciliary nerves in the horizontal meridian or when treating anterior to the equator.

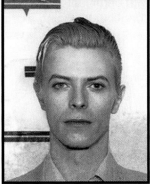

Figure 2. David Bowie's eyes.

You can bet that if your laser can affect iris function, it can also affect ciliary body function—and this can be far more annoying. A heavy PRP can definitely decrease accommodation. This is particularly important in a patient who is in the pre-presbyopic or early presbyopic age range. Remember that diabetics can have autonomic neuropathy to begin with, and if you tip them into more pronounced presbyopia, you can end up with a very unhappy patient, even if your superb laser has spared them from total blindness. Again, you have to do what you have to do, but it is important to both warn patients about this possibility so they are not surprised, and to try to go easy when treating over the nerves if possible.

There are also patients that can develop rather severe iritis after a laser. This is more likely with hot and heavy treatment, and sometimes it can even result in synechia formation—something to be avoided in patients that need to be dilated a lot to see the back of their eye. (Synechia can also occur of you are clipping the pupil margin with your treatment. This is more likely with an indirect ophthalmoscope delivery system, but it can happen with a slit lamp laser, too.) Consider using a topical steroid and cycloplegic if you put in a lot of laser or if you have a patient with a history of uveitis.

Patients can also have problems related to elevated intraocular pressure. Heavy panretinal photocoagulation can cause diminished outflow because of swelling of the ciliary body. Occasionally this swelling can even rotate the iris enough to cause angle-closure glaucoma. This is more likely in patients who already have narrow angles, and you may want to avoid very heavy treatment in one session with such patients. This is also something to keep in mind if you have a patient with longstanding glaucoma and fragile nerves. Even if they don't get angle closure they can have a transient rise in pressure that can threaten their nerve, and you should adjust your treatment accordingly.

The important thing is that if a patient calls you because of pain subsequent to panretinal photocoagulation, do not assume that they are a wimp and phone in some narcotics. You really should look at them to determine if they have developed uveitis, elevated pressure or even angle closure. By the way, these problems tended to be more common in the old days when patients were pounded with confluent white-hot laser burns or, worse, were treated with xenon photocoagulation. Doing a gradual, careful PRP is much less likely to result in problems, but it is still important to be aware of all the trouble you can cause.

POSTERIOR SEGMENT

Most posterior segment issues have already been discussed in the preceding chapters—but a little repetition is good, because you want to make it through your whole career without gaining personal experience with any of these problems.

Perhaps the most disastrous mistake is to create an inadvertent foveal burn. Follow all the advice about constantly checking your location in the fundus and *always* know for sure where you are. Remember that you are far more likely to do something like this when you start to feel very comfortable with your laser skills, and that it is especially likely to occur when you are frantically trying to stay above water on a busy clinic day. Don't ever get overconfident, and don't ever let yourself feel rushed when you are guiding coherent light into a fellow human being's eye. You don't want your handiwork to turn into a treasured slide in some retina specialist's talk on laser complications.

If you forget which eye you are treating, or if you mix up which side of the eye you are treating while using an indirect lens, you can easily get lost. This is especially likely when treating in the temporal aspect of the posterior pole, where there is no optic disc or vascular arcade to warn you that you are crossing into no man's land. This can happen more readily if your view is limited by a small pupil, or if media opacities interfere with your ability to sweep around and orient yourself. Also, remember that if you are using the large mirror in a Goldmann three mirror lens, it is possible to get deep into the macula without realizing it, especially if the patient is looking toward this mirror (Figure 3 in Chapter 4). Sometimes patients will have large vessels running across the posterior pole that can simulate the appearance of nasal retina, and this can really confuse you if you are not careful. If you come across such a patient, be *very* careful about where you are treating.

Almost all of these problems can be overcome by simply checking where you are at all times so that you do not get a chance to get lost. As mentioned before, it is good to set landmarks in your head so that if you see them, you know you are in a danger zone. Another option, especially when performing PRPs, is to put a line of laser spots at the posterior edge of your planned treatment pattern and then treat outward from this line—always moving from the back of the eye to the front—so at all times you are moving away from the posterior pole as you place spots.

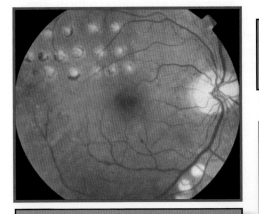

Figure 3. (Left) Whew, just in time. Five out of five doctors recommend not putting your PRP here...

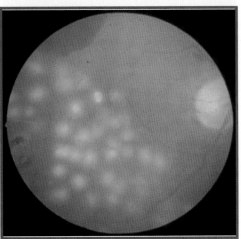

Figure 4. (Right) This should make your primary sexual organs shrivel. But you can see how easy it could be to do this, given the hazy view, the hemorrhage that obscures retinal vessels and the nearby laser scars. All of these things can make you think you are where you are not.

There are also a host of complications related to poor power management with your spot size and intensity. If you remember all of the variables that can get you into trouble, you can stay out of trouble. For instance, if you decrease the spot size, or if your aiming beam suddenly becomes smaller and brighter, you know you need to cut back on the power.

The point is that a hot spot can cause any number of problems, all of which are bad. A hot spot can cause a vitreous hemorrhage, intraretinal hemorrhage, subretinal hemorrhage, and even choroidal hemorrhage if you manage to burn down deeply. Remember, too, that if you have actually done any of these things, then you should keep pressure on the eye with the contact lens until any bleeding stops. Also remember that if you burned something bad enough to cause a hemorrhage, you have probably also created a full-thickness retinal hole. You want to make sure you treat around the offending area enough to tack the retina down so you don't get a detachment.

A severe burn in the peripheral retina can also result in a late complication known as a choroidal-vitreal anastamosis. In this case a hot burn gets so deep that choroidal vessels are induced to anastamose with retinal vessels and then the ensuing network grows up into the vitreous, creating very aggressive, destructive neovascularization. This problem was more likely in the bad old days, and often occurred when people were using very heavy treatment with laser or xenon arc in an attempt to directly shut down NVE. This is something that is useful to know about in the abstract, but you should never come close to causing it.

You can also poke holes in things without a hemorrhage, and this is particularly noticeable if you burn through Bruch's membrane while doing a focal. The sickening sight and sound of this, as mentioned in Chapter 8, is something you should strive to never experience. If it does happen, remember that such a spot may be nidus for development of a choroidal neovascular membrane, and you will want to watch for any unusual subretinal hemorrhage or localized macular edema that heralds the development of such a problem. Also, recall that you do not necessarily have to break Bruch's membrane to get a neovascular membrane; it can also occur around less intense laser treatment. All of this is why you should strive to do the least amount of laser necessary to treat macular edema.

Also remember that there are occasional patients who are extremely good observers and will notice each and every focal spot that you apply. These are more likely to be younger, type-A patients who do not have a lot of diabetic disease and who are much more likely to notice the punctate changes in their paramacular vision. As mentioned in the chapter on informed consent for treating diabetic macular edema, you want to make sure patients are aware of this possibility and you should always treat as lightly as you can—but if they need treatment, they need treatment.

There are also a few things that can happen when treating proliferative disease that are not really complications, but your patient may be likely to feel that they are—for instance, the occurrence of a vitreous hemorrhage shortly after a PRP due to the shrinkage of the blood vessels. There is really no way to avoid this, and it may actually represent a good response to treatment. However, you do need to warn the patient about this possibility, especially if they are presenting with asymptomatic proliferative disease.

The other "complication" is that the patient may develop more significant traction, perhaps even a retinal detachment, as the neovascular tissue responds to your treatment. If you think something like this might happen you want to be very clear about this prior to treatment, especially in patients who are presenting late in their proliferative career with extensive disease that should never have been allowed to develop in the first place. If you are worried that this could be a big problem, you might want to refer the patient to your friendly neighborhood retina specialist.

Sometimes a very aggressive PRP can result in an exudative retinal detachment and/or choroidal effusions, which can even simulate a rhegmatogenous retinal detachment. Usually, this problem is evidence of a very sick eye, and it is more likely to occur in patients who get lots of hot spots in one sitting. If you actually manage to do something like this to a patient, you should give them topical steroids and cycloplegics to help things settle down, and then try to be gentle with any additional treatment.

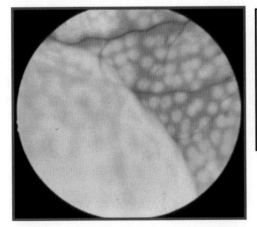

Figure 5. Intense PRP resulting in a peripheral serous retinal detachment. (Figures 1, 3 and 4 courtesy of James C. Folk, M.D. [the images—not the techniques])

There are other, stranger things that have been reported. For instance, patients have developed thermal optic neuritis from excessive treatment near the nerve, or retinal vasculitis and even vascular occlusion from hot burns on vessels. You should never, ever have any experience with entities such as this; they are included simply for completeness.

A more common problem associated with panretinal photocoagulation is peripheral field loss, and this was especially likely in the olden days when large amounts of laser were applied rapidly. Measurable changes can occur in up to 50% of patients, although milder treatment seems to have less of an effect.[1] Of course, patients are receiving the treatment in the first place because the bulk of their peripheral retina is either dead or dying off—the difference being that if they choose to have field loss from their disease alone, they have to accept the risk of total vision loss from untreated retinopathy. In other words, whether peripheral field loss is related to the disease or your treatment is largely academic; the patient really has no choice. Hopefully you, with your newly gleaned knowledge, will be able to put in a gentle yet effective PRP with less risk of dramatic visual field loss than was seen in the old days. Still, this can be a real problem—especially in terms of driving—and hopefully a time will come when patients won't have to risk this additional insult to their vision as new pharmacologic treatments come online.

Panretinal photocoagulation can also cause problems with dark adaptation, nyctalopia and color vision, all of which seem more likely with heavier treatments. However, it is hard to know to what degree these can be attributed to the laser versus the severity of the underlying retinopathy. Even diabetics who do not need PRP complain of problems along these lines as they get older and experience the general deterioration of retinal function that occurs with the disease. Nevertheless, if significant problems occur right after a laser, then it probably was the laser and patients need to be warned about this possibility.

A related problem is the fact that many diabetics will complain of increased sensitivity to light. Again, this may represent overall generalized deterioration due to diabetes. However, it is also likely that the loss of peripheral pigmentation that accompanies extensive scarring from laser treatment allows light to bounce around in the eye, so that the remaining compromised retina has even more problems in bright light situations.

Of course, one of the main complications of both macular treatment and PRP is decreased central visual acuity. This is usually due to exacerbation of pre-existing macular edema, and ways to avoid this are specifically covered in the chapters on performing these treatments.

ONE LAST COMPLICATION

After having carefully reviewed all the different ways you can screw up with lasers, it is important to remember that perhaps one of the most worrisome complications is to have your treatment fail because it was inadequate. Generally, a "less is more" technique is the best way to go, because the fewer spots you need to place—for any treatment—the more vision your patient gets to keep. Unfortunately, if you don't put in enough spots to control the disease, then you for sure haven't done the patient any favors. Decisions about how aggressive to be will become easier with time and experience, but remember, if you do end up going light with any laser, watch the patient closely and do not allow them to be lost to follow up for any reason.

References and Suggested Reading

1.   Fong DS, Girach A, Boney A. Visual side effects of successful scatter laser photocoagulation surgery for proliferative diabetic retinopathy: a literature review. Retina 2007;27:816-24.

2.   Folk JC, Pulido JS. Laser photocoagulation of the retina and choroid. San Francisco: American Academy of Ophthalmology, 1997.

Singerman LJ, Coscas GJ. Current techniques in ophthalmic laser surgery, 3rd ed. Boston: Butterworth-Heineman, 1999.

L'Esperance FA. Ophthalmic lasers, 3rd ed. St. Louis: Mosby, 1989.

Bloom, SM, Brucker, AJ. Laser Surgery of the Posterior Segment. Philadelphia: Lippincott Williams & Wilkins, 1997.

Davis MD, Blodi BA. Proliferative Diabetic Retinopathy. In: Ryan SJ. Retina, 4th ed. Philadelphia: Elsevier Mosby, 2006:v.2, pp 1285-1322.

Blondeau P, Pavan PR, Phelps CD. Acute pressure elevation following panretinal photocoagulation. Arch Ophthalmol 1981;99:1239-41.

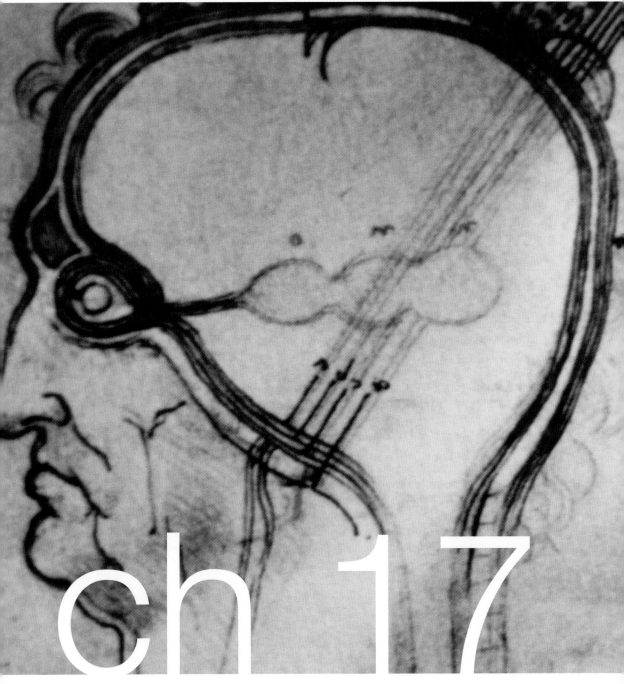

ch 17

Now What?
Following up a PRP and All Those Little Hemorrhages

One of the most difficult aspects of treating proliferative diabetic retinopathy is deciding whether further treatment is warranted. About two thirds to three fourths of treated eyes will demonstrate regression, and sometimes this can begin as early as a few days after treatment. It usually takes a bit longer to see the full effect of the laser, so it is common to check patients at about six to eight weeks after the last laser session to get a sense their response. If there is a potential for significant traction or if the patient is particularly worrisome, it makes sense to see them sooner.

The ideal response is complete resolution of the neovascularization, period. Unfortunately, this ideal is not as common as one would wish, especially in younger patients, and often there are persistent vessels of some sort. If there is any sense that the vessels are growing, or if there is evidence of vitreous hemorrhaging (even small amounts of blood in the far periphery that are otherwise asymptomatic), then it is very reasonable to put in more laser. Although there are no controlled studies defining the amount of laser, there is a sense that if the first treatment does not work, a rather substantial amount of laser is necessary to generate any sort of useful response the second time around. For instance, it probably does not help to put in 200 to 300 spots in a patient with persistent disease—instead, it seems that such patients usually need an additional critical mass of perhaps 500 to 1,000 spots.[1] The exception to this would be if there is an area of the fundus that has less treatment, and especially if the new vessels are clearly growing in the direction of the untreated area. In this case, a smaller amount of treatment directed to the ischemic area may be all you need.

As mentioned before, you can squeeze in over 6,000 spots to control the disease, but such patients may benefit from referral for intravitreal therapy and/or a vitrectomy, rather than dribbling in more and more laser over several months and slowly eliminating all their visual field. The vitreous does seem to play a role in stimulating the blood vessels, and by having it removed patients may get by with much less laser. Chapter 18 discusses when to consider referral in more depth.

If the blood vessels seem to have shrunk back somewhat, but have not disappeared, the decision to treat can be more difficult. Some patients may simply have persistent neovascularization that doesn't cause trouble for years, and for these patients additional laser is a waste of time and peripheral vision. If the residual vessels are small in size and have really shrunk down in caliber, and if they are not widespread, it makes sense to watch them a bit. Another pattern that suggests quiescence is if the tips of the vessels have receded into thick, clublike endings.

If the vessels are becoming more fibrotic in nature it suggests that the retinopathy is leaving the proliferative phase and laser may not be needed (but do watch for progressive traction). On the other hand, if the tips of the vessels consist of fine, sprouting buds, then treatment should be added. Sometimes a fluorescein angiogram can be helpful—active vessels can be very leaky, whereas quiescent, involuted vessels will leak much less.

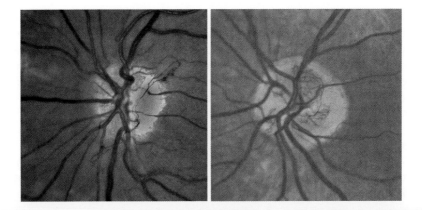

Figure 1. Old and new neovascularization. The photo on the left shows the kind of thready, ropy appearance of regressed neo after PRP. Note the clumpy, grapelike appearance of the ends of the vessels; they have shriveled up in failure. The photo on the right shows active vessels. Note how they are spread out and arborized, with fine vessels at the tips growing in all directions. Also note that the image on the left was Photoshop'd to make the vessels easier to see. (Right photo courtesy of the Early Treatment Diabetic Retinopathy Study Group)

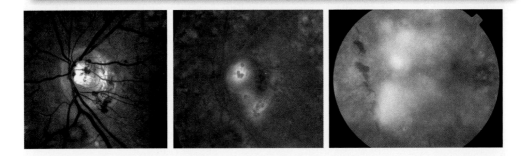

Figure 2. Another example of regressed neovascularization, showing the shriveled appearance of the old vessels. Note the relative lack of staining in the later phases of the angiogram (middle). Such vessels are often nicely backlit by the small amount of fluorescein that does leak out. Compare this to the figure on the right, which shows the florid leakage seen with new, active vessels: There is no view whatsoever of the actual vessels themselves, because they are obscured by all the fluorescence.

Another important variable is the density of your PRP. If you were trying to go lightly and the vessels don't seem to be regressing, then you should consider filling in the PRP pattern. An angiogram may be helpful here because it may demonstrate areas of non-perfusion that are not obvious clinically and you can see whether your initial laser covered such areas.

If you do decide to add treatment, you can fill in between spots and extend your treatment further into the periphery. You can also extend the treatment closer to the center of the macula, but if you really think you need to laser valuable real estate, you may want to get a second opinion beforehand. Also, if you need to treat over previously treated retina you need to be very careful about where you place your spots. Treatment that hits previous laser scars may be painful for the patient, and more importantly, the cicatricial pigmentation can dramatically increase the laser uptake and cause a hemorrhage or hole.

Other factors that may help you decide about how hard to treat residual vessels were discussed in preceding chapters. They include the patient's age, the course of the fellow eye, the degree of compliance and control, and whether the patient is on Coumadin.

A **conundrum** that occasionally comes up is when a patient had the first stage of a PRP performed, but either never returned for follow up or the treating physician was happy with the initial results and did no further treatment. You may see these patients years later with partially treated neovascularization, no symptoms, and laser treatment in only one sector of the fundus. If they have been stable for quite some time, and if they have good systemic control, it is reasonable to observe them. There is a risk of progression of their proliferative disease if they are left untreated, but there is also a risk of converting a happy asymptomatic patient into a bitterly symptomatic patient from problems related to a full dose of PRP. You just have to use your clinical judgment, and if the patient does elect observation it is important that they understand the risks and the need for continuous follow up.

The converse occurs when a previously untreated patient needs treatment and has only a single clump of neovascularization in one part of the fundus.* It may seem that doing laser in only that area is all that is needed. This is not a good idea. A localized area of neovascularization does not mean that only one part of the retina is ischemic; there are no secret barricades to vasoproliferative substances in the eye. You may be able to get away with a milder PRP in such a patient, but once a patient crosses the line into needing laser, it is a good idea to treat all around the fundus rather than in one local area.

*By the way, make sure you have the correct diagnosis in such a patient. For instance, they could have the entity mentioned in Chapter 26 that begins with a "B."

It turns out that in addition to figuring out how to manage residual neovascularization, there can also be problems deciding what to do about patients who have recurrent vitreous hemorrhages. It turns out that it is not uncommon for diabetics with persistent neovascularization to have intermittent hemorrhages over the years. If the vessels are growing or appear succulent, and there are significant areas of untreated retina, then adding more PRP is the simplest thing to do.

Sometimes, however, hemorrhages may be due to intrinsic vascular fragility; an eye that is full of beat-up old blood vessels will have an occasional spontaneous hemorrhage, just like people can have spontaneous bruises on their legs. More laser is unlikely to make any difference in such patients, and if you feel their proliferative disease is burned out and their PRP pattern is adequate, then observation is all that is needed.

A more common problem is age-related vitreous contraction beginning to tug at old neovascularization. In fact, patients may go years with nicely controlled disease, and then suddenly start to get hemorrhages simply because they have survived long enough for their vitreous to shrink and start pulling on the regressed vessels. Adding more laser may be irrelevant for such patients, because now a mechanical problem is being imposed on their otherwise quiescent proliferative disease. On the other hand, it may be reasonable to fill in with more laser if there are large areas of untreated retina in the periphery (the assumption would be that vasoproliferative factors released by the untreated retina are keeping the vessels a bit more swollen than they might otherwise be, and they are therefore more likely to hemorrhage with even a little traction). Usually, however, such patients will need a vitrectomy if the hemorrhages are recurrent and do not clear quickly.

A variation on this theme is if the patient begins to develop vitreous contraction, and then is fortunate enough to get a complete vitreous separation from the retina. If this happens, patients almost always get a vitreous hemorrhage, but the process also eliminates all the traction. These patients may have very little in the way of subsequent hemorrhaging, and there is no role for more laser.

And once again: Although complete vitreous separation is usually a cause for celebration in the setting of diabetic retinopathy, don't forget to look carefully for retinal breaks or tears.

However, a total vitreous detachment is a lucky event that does not happen too often; usually the vitreous is only partially separated, and it then applies even greater traction wherever it remains attached. If there are areas where the PRP pattern is light, then more laser may help to shrink down the vessels that are now being tugged on more aggressively. Usually a vitrectomy is required if the hemorrhaging is persistent.

If there is one patch of neovascularization that keeps bleeding in spite of good laser, some doctors advocate attempting to directly close the offending vessels with focal laser. This may be something to try if the vessels are small and flat and the retina is relatively healthy—but this is something that is much easier said than done even in the best of circumstances. If the vessels are big or elevated, or if the retina is thin and on stretch, you can end up creating a hole which will cause a detachment. This is a big disaster. If you really want to try this technique, consider getting some help before you do—nowadays a vitrectomy is probably safer.

ODDS & ENDS

How soon do you bring in a diabetic with symptoms from a hemorrhage?

Traditionally, any patient with a sudden change in floaters needs same-day service to rule out a retinal tear. Because diabetics may have off-and-on hemorrhaging for years, and because such symptoms rarely indicate an acute problem like a retinal tear or detachment, there is a tendency to bend this rule.

In an ideal world, it would be best to get everyone in quickly just to be safe. It will relieve the patient's anxiety, and you may occasionally have a chance to get some laser in before a hemorrhage spreads around, or you may rarely find something unexpected like a retinal tear. Practically speaking, however, if you have a lot of diabetic patients you could bring your practice to a standstill trying to get everyone in immediately—something that is usually not necessary for patients who have already had occasional hemorrhages and who have long-standing disease that is otherwise well controlled. You will even find that diabetics who have intermittent hemorrhages will ask you if it is okay to *not* call when they have a hemorrhage so they don't have to keep coming in all the time.*

All these symptomatic patients can create a rather difficult dilemma that is not fully addressed in the literature. Although the safest approach is to get everyone in as soon as they call, at times doctors will compromise by bringing them in within a few days. This allows the hemorrhage to clear a bit and also prevents a totally overbooked schedule—something that can lead to a different set of quality-of-care problems. You must understand, however, that although this is a rationalization retina doctors feel comfortable with, there is always a chance of missing something acute.

Ultimately, deciding whether to get a diabetic with vitreous hemorrhage symptoms in immediately is a function of several variables. One important factor is the level of panic on the part of the patient (you should always try to get a freaked-out patient in quickly, even if you don't think anything is going on—it is both nicer and safer). Other factors include whether this is their first hemorrhage or one of many, how well you know the patient's retinopathy and the patient's ability to accurately convey the symptoms over the phone (i.e., is their vision diffusely hazy but intact—implying a hemorrhage—or do they have a dense black shadow in one area, suggesting a detachment?). A final factor is how much

---

* Even though it is reasonable for a patient with well controlled disease and a history of intermittent hemorrhages to "wait it out and call only if it gets worse," it is probably not a good idea for you to actually suggest this. If the patient turns out to be the rare one who has a "routine" hemorrhage and then has their retina fall off because they waited before calling, you will feel very bad and their attorney will feel very good. It may be best to simply tell them the risk of not calling—small though it may be—and then let them decide what they want to do. It turns out that most diabetic patients who are used to having occasional hemorrhages will wait them out anyway.

sleep you will lose if you postpone the evaluation for a day or so. The choice will be yours.

What about the effect of physical activity on hemorrhages?

Almost all patients assume that any sort of lifting or straining just has to make the little blood vessels in their eyes pop open. It turns out that it is very unusual for a diabetic patient to routinely hemorrhage due to physical activity; usually, hemorrhages occur during sleep or rest.[2] As a result, patients are not normally given any sort of restrictions. This is important because it allows them to pursue a normal life that includes vigorous exercise and other activities that are beneficial to their diabetic control and overall health. You may want to mention this specifically, even if they don't ask, because some patients will simply assume they should restrict their activity (or their family members may restrict it for them).

You may come across rare patients in whom straining will contribute to hemorrhaging, and usually these patients will be able to give a very consistent history indicating an association. These patients may need more laser or even a vitrectomy, although sometimes simply waiting it out allows the vessels to become fibrotic and the problem goes away.

Finally, there are times when a patient with old, quiescent proliferative disease will hemorrhage after an episode of coughing or vomiting, or perhaps after some sort of trauma. At times a hemorrhage can occur after an insulin reaction. If the retinopathy is stable, these events tend to be self-limited and are unlikely to require additional treatment.

Here is one other useful tip when caring for patients with proliferative disease—or for patients with any form of retinopathy, for that matter. You should always point out at the end of your exam that retinopathy can be very unpredictable, and that although a patient may appear stable in the office they need to understand that something unexpected could happen anytime—even that evening. If you take care of enough diabetics you will have one or two of them call back with a hemorrhage within a day of an exam wherein you pronounced them "clean." It is quite easy for them to think that you missed something when, in fact, there was nothing to treat and the blame lies with unpredictable changes in their vitreo-retinal interface. Once again, it is always better if you warn a patient about something before it happens. (Of course, if you *did* miss something, this can be a great way to cover yourself—but hopefully this will never be your primary reason for mentioning this.)

References and Suggested Reading

1.   Davis MD, Blodi BA. Proliferative Diabetic Retinopathy. In: Ryan SJ. Retina, 4th ed. Philadelphia: Elsevier Mosby, 2006:v.2, pp 1285-1322.

2.   Anderson B, Jr. Activity and diabetic vitreous hemorrhages. Ophthalmology 1980;87:173-5.

Folk JC, Pulido JS. Laser photocoagulation of the retina and choroid. San Francisco: American Academy of Ophthalmology, 1997.

Singerman LJ, Coscas GJ. Current techniques in ophthalmic laser surgery, 3rd ed. Boston: Butterworth-Heineman, 1999.

Bloom, SM, Brucker, AJ. Laser Surgery of the Posterior Segment. Philadelphia: Lippincott Williams & Wilkins, 1997.

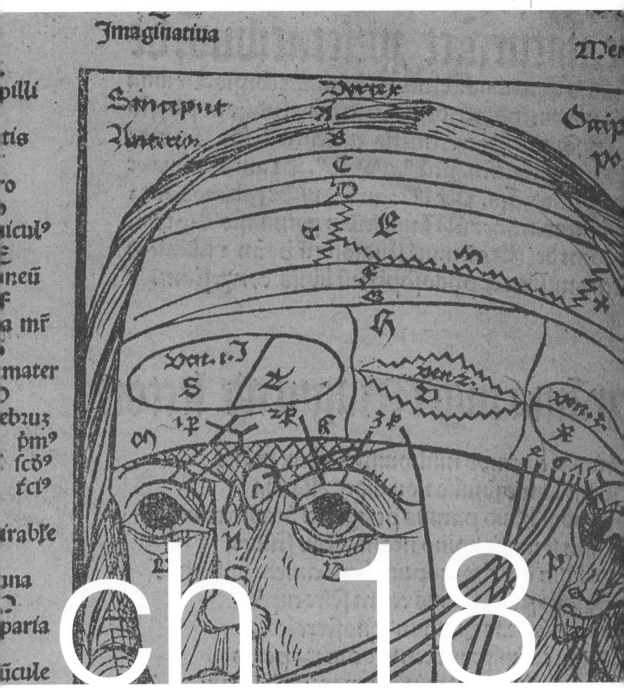

ch 18

When to Bail Out, Give Up, Drop Off the Key, Lee, and Refer for Vitrectomy

Vitrectomy has dramatically changed the prognosis for many patients with severe proliferative diabetic retinopathy. It definitely ain't Hollywood, though— the level of expectation that goes along with cataract surgery does not apply to vitrectomies. Although patients with routine non-clearing vitreous hemorrhages tend to do very well, patients with more aggressive neovascular traction can be disappointed with the results of even very successful surgery. It is also important to remember that vitrectomy can have significant complications, and these complications are more likely in sicker eyes. A nicely reattached retina may just not work because it is dead, or an ischemic diabetic eye may unavoidably fold up into neovascular glaucoma after perfect surgery. You cannot have patients thinking that a quick trip to the vitrectomy shop will solve things lickety-split.

One never quite knows which diabetic eye will be the one that will fall apart after surgery, and it is this ever-present risk that tends to make retinal surgeons a bit conservative. This is a very different mindset from cataract surgery or Lasik, which are performed more readily because they carry a smaller risk of complications and because experience tells you that the patient is likely to be happy with the result. In fact, the best way to do a vitrectomy is to avoid it altogether with aggressive control of the patient's systemic vascular risk factors, aggressive follow up, and appropriate photocoagulation. Unfortunately, in spite of all the king's horses, etc., there are patients who cannot be controlled with laser alone, and it is great that many heroic pioneers developed vitrectomy surgery so that we can save many of these downward-spiraling eyes. You just have to know when the time is right to refer.

Non-clearing Vitreous Hemorrhages

The traditional indication for vitrectomy is a non-clearing vitreous hemorrhage. The exact timing of surgery is variable. It would be great if you could just memorize one number, but there is no "automatic" time to operate. There are guaranteed risks with surgery; vitrectomy carries about a 2 to 5% complication rate, and that number goes up in eyes that are sicker or out of control. On the other hand, doing nothing can also be risky because you can't see the retina to be sure it is safe from problems such as macular edema or a progressive traction detachment. The real issue is deciding at what time the risks of observation become worse than the risk of intervention. Perhaps the most important factor is how aggressive the patient's retinopathy happens to be.

Older patients tend to have more quiescent disease, and they may have long-standing vitreous hemorrhages without developing any irreversible problems. For these patients, it may be reasonable to wait at least three to four months to allow for clearing. For some elderly patients, the thought of having surgery is way worse than a blurry eye, and so they may want to wait even longer.

However, most retina folks start to get a little itchy when no one has seen the retina after a three- to four-month time frame, even for these relatively calm eyes, because there is always a chance that edema or traction not seen with a B-scan could be sneaking up on the fovea. In other words, even if the patient is content to wait they need to understand that the three- to four-month time frame is about when the progressive risk of unobserved retinal damage gradually begins to outweigh the fixed risk of surgery. This does not mean they *have* to have surgery; it just means that you need to convey the shifting of the risk-to-benefit scales. Note that some patients will not give you the chance to wait things out like this—having all that junk sloshing around in their vision is very disturbing, and you might as well refer them earlier because they are unlikely to listen to you anyway.

By the way, if you are going to observe many of these patients on your own, you really need to have access to a B-scan to be certain that everything is OK while you wait. It is risky to follow patients if you cannot be reasonably certain that the retina is where it is supposed to be. How often should they be checked? There is no definite answer, but most of the time it is safe to monitor patients about once a month. This does not give the eye a lot of time to mess itself up between visits. (Remember that the patient may not be able to tell if they are getting a retinal detachment because they don't have enough vision to notice a change.) If the hemorrhage is mild or clearing, the patient may not need to be seen as often. Patients should also be reminded to call immediately if they think their vision is getting noticeably worse or if the eye is getting red and painful (i.e., neovascular or hemolytic glaucoma).

Although the three- to four-month rule can work for benign hemorrhages in otherwise calm eyes, there are other patients who may need to be encouraged to move more rapidly towards surgery. This is especially true in younger patients with more aggressive disease, and trebly true if the patient has an eye full of blood but has not had a chance to get a full laser treatment. These patients should be considered for early vitrectomy, perhaps within a month of presenting, in order to avoid tractional problems that arise as the blood vessels continue to slowly grow unobserved beneath the hemorrhage. Sometimes, these patients will have dense premacular hemorrhages, such that the blood is loculated in front of the posterior pole. Although you can still see a lot of the peripheral retina in such an eye, it is felt that there is a significant risk of progressive fibrovascular growth and traction and that early vitrectomy is warranted. (FYI: Sometimes these patients can benefit from YAG puncture of the loculated hemorrhage in order to allow it to spread out and dissolve. This is not done commonly—and the technique is well beyond the scope of this book—but it does come in handy on occasion.)

Another brief pep talk for you and the patient you are referring:
Sometimes patients think that if you are referring them out it is a sure indication that all those lasers that you hammered in (and billed them for) didn't do anything. It is worth pointing out that sending the patient off to the retina world is a clear-cut sign that the lasers have saved the eye—without the laser to reverse the eye's suicidal tendencies, the retina would have crumpled up a long time ago and there would be no vision whatsoever to save. What the laser cannot do, however, is to reverse vitreous traction on the patient's blood vessels. Emphasize that the patient now has a largely mechanical problem that needs steel, not more of Planck's constant, and that the laser has worked well enough to get them safely to the point of referral. A good retina specialist will make this point for you when the patient is first seen—but it helps for the patient to hear it on both ends of the consultation.

Another factor that may influence the decision to operate is whether the patient has specific visual needs that require rapid recovery. Some patients are willing to take the risk of surgery quickly, just to try to get better faster for professional or personal reasons. Such patients need to be reminded, however, that the recovery from a vitrectomy can be much more unpredictable than the recovery from anterior segment surgery. For instance, if the patient needs a gas bubble for any reason, or if there is a post-op hemorrhage, their visual recovery can be rather slow. The point is that although your friendly neighborhood retina specialist will go over this fully with the patient, you should not promise your patients a fast, easy recovery when you refer them because you will jinx them for sure.

A final "hemorrhagic" reason to have surgery can occur in patients who have well controlled proliferative disease, yet continue to have recurrent mild hemorrhages from involuted vessels. Such hemorrhages can drive a patient nuts as they come and go, even if the hemorrhages clear and the vision is good between episodes. There is no definite number of hemorrhages that merits surgery; some patients will put up with only a few, while others will have a hemorrhage every few months for years before asking for surgery. Because these patients are more "elective" than the typical diabetic who needs a vitrectomy it is especially important that they understand the risks and benefits.

Other Indications

There are some other indications for vitrectomy besides a non-clearing vitreous hemorrhage, and most of these are fairly obvious. For instance, referral is mandatory if the patient appears to be developing progressive traction that is threatening the macula, or if the macula has just been yanked off. Sometimes, however, making this call is not as easy as one would think. The traction can build up very slowly, often simulating refractory macular edema as the retina is slowly thickened—like a peanut butter and jelly sandwich being pulled open. If you are not sure about the stability based on your clinical exam, an OCT can be very helpful assuming care is taken to maintain uniform fixation between tests.

Don't depend entirely on technology, though. You can always resort to ancient and primitive methods, such as actually talking to the patient about their symptoms. Slowly progressive traction can cause metamorphopsia or changes in peripheral vision that patients can detect, and you should take complaints along these lines very seriously, even if you cannot see any clinically apparent changes. Sometimes it helps to provide patients with an Amsler grid to help them monitor for progression. If there is any doubt, a referral is in order. This is because the results of surgery in this situation tend to be much better if the problem is fixed before the fovea pops off. (Of course, your retina person then has to weigh the risks of doing surgery that may snuff out vision versus losing vision from conservative observation—but that is why he or she did a fellowship in the first place.)

On the other hand, sometimes ominous-looking traction can be quite stable. In fact, the majority of patients with localized areas of traction do not progress. At times the retina can even look like a campground full of hammocks and pup-tents, yet the patient never needs surgery. A very creepy pattern can occasional-ly develop because many so-called diabetic traction retinal detachments are, in fact, areas of tractional retinoschisis—there is still an outer layer of retina stuck to the RPE. These eyes can sometimes get nasty-looking inner-layer holes that resemble Swiss cheese draped over clotheslines, leaving one wondering how on earth the retina is remaining attached at all. (It remains in place, of course, be-cause there are no true full-thickness holes.) Monitoring, and especially lasering, eyes filled with traction can be a bit nuanced and usually such eyes are referred to specialists until they are known to be stable. If you are watching eyes like this, make sure the patients know when to call.

Retinas can become so atrophic, however, that they do develop full-thickness holes, and then patients get a rhegmatogenous detachment in addition to any traction that is present. The rather dramatic downturn in their vision and the floppy, bulbous appearance of the retina usually make the need for referral obvi-ous. Putting an atrophic, lasered-out retina back on the RPE and getting it to stay there can be difficult, to say the least, and the visual outcomes—although better than nothing—do not tend to be great. Please don't pat such a patient on the back and say that they will be as good as new after surgery.

Another indication for vitrectomy is the presence of progressive rubeosis in the setting of a vitreous hemorrhage that precludes laser treatment. In the old days, people would try to put in panretinal cryotherapy without visualizing the retina, trying to kill off enough retina to stop the neovascularization and give the eye a chance to clear the hemorrhage. This approach may still be used if a patient is too sick for surgery or if you do not have access to a vitreoretinal specialist. If there is a chance of useful vision being obtained from the eye, however, it is best to do a vitrectomy rather than "blind" cryotherapy; cryo can really stir up pain, inflammation and scarring, and is more of a last-resort approach. Intravitreal anti-VEGF treatment can be invaluable in this situation, as well. Basically, pa-tients who have progressive anterior segment neovascularization and a vitreous hemorrhage should receive a prompt referral.

Another less common reason for performing a vitrectomy is elevated in-traocular pressure secondary to the presence of vitreous blood coming into the anterior chamber and clogging up the trabecular meshwork. This process can actually occur in three ways:

1. Fresh erythrocytes accumulating in the meshwork.
2. Hemolytic glaucoma, wherein hemosiderin-filled macrophages obstruct the meshwork.
3. Ghost cell glaucoma, wherein erythrocytes lose their hemoglobin and block the meshwork because they are less pliable than normal erythrocytes. Such cells are khaki-colored and are usually seen with old, yellowish vitreous blood.

Whatever the pathology, the pressure can get quite high, and if it does not re-spond to medical management a vitrectomy is required to wash the eye out.

There is another group of patients that would likely benefit from early referral: the ones who respond poorly to PRP—even if a hemorrhage has not yet occurred. These tend to be younger Type 1 diabetics with a history of non-compliance, and it is hard to specify the exact level of disease that merits referral. Like the line about knowing the difference between art and pornography, however, you will recognize such patients when you see them. Anytime vascular fronds fail to respond to a solid PRP, you can assume you are dealing with an eye that is hell-bent on destroying itself and you generally do not want your name to be the last one on the chart.

One option for these patients is to keep hammering in laser from the arcade to the ora, but this may just destroy peripheral visual field without controlling the problem—recall that the vessels are locked onto the vitreous and supping on the vasoproliferative substances that reside there because the eye is diffusely ischemic. The decision whether to operate on such patients is complicated; they tend to have relatively preserved vision, and the risks are not small. The point is that if your laser is not slowing down the growth of new vessels, it is better to get an early consult than to wait for multiple lasers to not work and then refer in a patient with big vessels, traction detachments and a totally atrophic peripheral retina, all of which carry a more guarded prognosis with surgery.

Refractory macular edema due to traction is another indication that may respond to a vitrectomy. Obvious cases usually have an epiretinal membrane that is gently tugging on the fovea and keeping the retina swollen. Sometimes the cortical vitreous can remain diffusely attached to the entire posterior pole, causing edema as it contracts without the presence of a distinct epiretinal membrane. This can sometimes appear as glistening sheen on the surface of the retina. OCT has really helped to identify situations where traction is contributing to the edema—this is also discussed in Chapter 10.

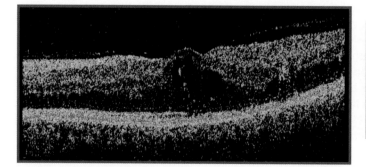

Figure 1. OCT demonstrating very subtle traction contributing to cystoid macular edema.

The role of vitrectomy for macular edema is less defined if there is no obvious epiretinal membrane or vitreous traction. There does not seem to be a lot of evidence that performing a vitrectomy in this setting is consistently effective, although there may be some patients who benefit from it. Studies are under way to try to define the role of vitrectomy in this situation, so hopefully there will be specific guidelines soon.

However, given all the potential treatments—including intravitreal therapy—anyone with bad macular edema should be referred whether it is for a vitrectomy or not. Remember that you can make two people happy with cataract surgery in the time it takes to explain treatments for refractory macular edema to one patient. Your unfixable problem is the retina person's reason for being, and retina specialists actually like doing it.

A more obscure reason to consider vitrectomy is the presence of vitreopapil-lary traction.[1] Sometimes the vitreous can be freed from the posterior pole but can still exert traction at the nerve. This is a fairly common configuration; many diabetics with burned-out proliferative disease will have sclerotic vascular fronds that emanate from the nerve and are tugged up into the vitreous. Occasionally, there is actually enough traction that the nerve fiber layer is slowly choked and vision is lost. These patients have progressive visual field defects and worsening central vision without any obvious cause such as a hemorrhage or direct foveal traction. This problem is relatively uncommon, but it should at least be kept in mind when treating patients who have a lot of traction yanking on the nerve.

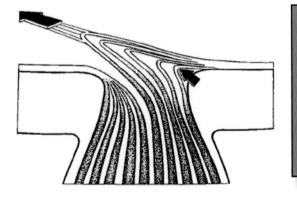

Figure 2. Schematic drawing of how traction at the nerve can damage the axons. Not a very common cause at all, but a good reminder of all the ways things can go wrong inside an eye. (Kroll P, Wiegand W, Schmidt J. Vitreopapillary traction in proliferative diabetic vitreoretinopathy. Br J Ophthalmol 1999;83:261-4.)

Finally, when it comes to performing a vitrectomy, whether for proliferative disease or macular edema, the path taken by the patient's fellow eye may help decide the issue. For instance, one would be much more inclined to do a vitrectomy if the fellow eye developed vision loss because a vitrectomy was not done soon enough. Conversely, a failed vitrectomy in one eye will make a patient very reluctant to have any surgery in the remaining eye—although this is usually the retina specialist's problem and not yours. Your job is to get the patient's disease as controlled as you can, and if things are not looking good then get them to a retina specialist at the appropriate time, and ideally a bit sooner, so that surgery can be considered when it can do the most good.

References and Suggested Reading

Gunduz K, Bakri SJ. Management of proliferative diabetic retinopathy. Compr Ophthalmol Update 2007;8:245-56.

Fong DS, Ferris FL. Practical Management of Diabetic Retinopathy. American Academy of Ophthalmology Focal Points 2003;21.

Early vitrectomy for severe vitreous hemorrhage in diabetic retinopathy. Four-year results of a randomized trial: Diabetic Retinopathy Vitrectomy Study Report 5. Arch Ophthalmol 1990;108:958-64.

Fraser-Bell S, Kaines A, Hykin PG. Update on treatments for diabetic macular edema. Curr Opin Ophthalmol 2008;19:185-9.

Davis MD, Blodi BA. Proliferative Diabetic Retinopathy. In: Ryan SJ. Retina, 4th ed. Philadelphia: Elsevier Mosby, 2006:v.2, pp 1285-1322.

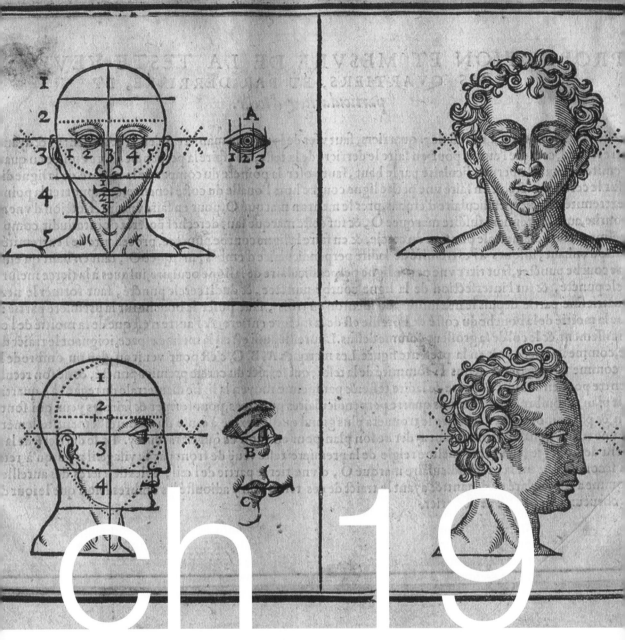

tions & mesures de la teste veuë de front, & de costé ou profil, & particularitez d

ch 19

Front End Trouble—Iris Neovascularization

Iris neovascularization is another form of proliferative diabetic retinopathy, and it usually indicates a very sick eye. First of all, though, do not be fooled by findings that may mimic true neovascularization. For instance, if you look carefully, you will often see tiny, reddish globular vessels on the pupil margin, especially if you study the iris prior to dilation in older diabetics. These vascular tufts may increase in number over time, but they do not usually cause any of the problems associated with true anterior segment neovascularization.

Another process that can simulate neovascularization is the development of iris atrophy, which can occur in patients with long-standing diabetes. This can result in increased visibility of normal iris vessels, especially in light-colored irides. The fact that such vessels are within the substance of the iris, and that they follow the normal iris architecture, will distinguish them from true neovascularization.

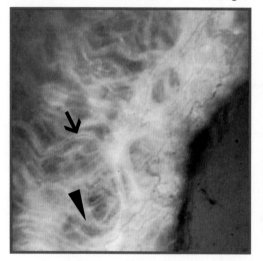

Figure 1. An example of iris neovascularization. The arrow points to a dilated yet normal vessel coursing with the iris stroma. This can simulate neovascularization, but is visible simply due to stromal atrophy. The rest of the vessels are arborizing over the surface of the iris, and are clearly abnormal. Note the puddle of blood loculated in an iris crypt (arrowhead). (Courtesy of Wallace L.M. Alward, M.D.)

However, if you see vessels arborizing on the surface of the iris—or if there is any neovascularization of the angle—then you are dealing with the real thing. This type of anterior segment proliferative retinopathy is usually an end-stage phenomenon that shows up well after problems have already occurred in the back of the eye. Diabetics start with proliferative diabetic retinopathy in the posterior segment and as the eye becomes progressively ischemic, vessels develop in the anterior segment, often in spite of previously adequate laser treatment.

Occasional patients, however, may develop anterior segment neovascularization without any evidence of posterior segment neovascularization—so always look at the iris closely before it is dilated. It can be really awkward if you tell a patient they are fine, yet they show up shortly thereafter with neovascular glaucoma— and then everyone in the clinic is wondering exactly how carefully you looked at the iris before diving into your 90-D exam.

Just because nothing is simple, there are even case reports of patients developing angle neovascularization without evidence of iris neovascularization.[1] Does this mean that you should be doing screening gonioscopy on every diabetic at every visit? In a perfect world, the answer to this question might be yes, but as a practical matter there is little chance that one could do this. The odds of finding something are very small, and the time involved (and the risk of scruffing up a bunch of diabetic epithelial cells) makes this approach impractical. Or, at least that is one possible rationalization--you are free to develop your own approach.

If you end up being like most folks, who do not automatically gonio everyone, you should still remember that isolated angle neovascularization is a possibility. It will serve to remind you that everything we do is a compromise on some level; by choosing not to do gonioscopy on all diabetics, someone, somewhere may get burned. At least try to think of this if a diabetic shows up with a pressure that is higher than their usual range.

A related issue is the way retina specialists often have their patients dilated without examining the iris first. This is also an inevitable compromise, but as a conscientious, comprehensive ophthalmologist, you are above this because you actually look at your patients well before they are dilated. If you are worried about something in the anterior segment that may not be seen after dilation, you need to make sure you let your retina specialist know in advance.

By the way, if a patient has vessels growing in the front part of the eye you should consider obtaining carotid Dopplers. The concern is that such patients may be developing global ocular ischemia from carotid disease superimposed on typical diabetic small-vessel disease. Dopplers are particularly important in a patient who develops anterior segment neovascularization without any posterior neovascularization—these patients may be more likely to have large-vessel disease. Finally, you should try to remember that there are other things that can cause new vessels to sprout in the anterior segment, such as uveitis or venous occlusive disease hiding behind diabetic retinopathy. These entities require very different diagnostic and therapeutic interventions. Never trust a diabetic eye to do anything predictably.

If you do pick up a case of diabetic anterior segment neovascularization, it is reassuring to know that it tends to evolve into neovascular glaucoma more slowly than neovascularization associated with, for instance, central retinal vein occlusions or ocular ischemia. In fact, not all diabetic anterior segment neovascularization will automatically turn into neovascular glaucoma; occasional patients can go for some time without getting a pressure rise.[2] However, it is generally considered risky to do nothing when faced with vessels on the iris—best to assume the worst and treat.

This "neovascular indolence" is important because it often means you may gain some flexibility with your PRP. Rather than firing in 2,000 fast spots, as you might do for rapidly progressive angle neovascularization with a central retinal vein occlusion, you can often do the laser in a divided dose to try to minimize the risk of blowing out the macula. These patients will still need a faster and more aggressive PRP than typical posterior segment proliferative disease; one can often prevail by putting in 800 to 1,000 spots at first, and then repeating the treatment in a week. More aggressive disease calls for more aggressive treatment with higher numbers, especially if the pressure is elevated.

Things get tricky if you identify the neovascularization, but the patient does not have any symptoms. Things get really tricky if they have a fragile macula. Under these circumstances, it is good to know that the neovascularization tends to progress slowly and you can at least try to start out with a slower PRP to spare the macula. Watch the patient carefully, though—at least once a week. If the vessels grow faster than your PRP is being placed, you will simply need to hit the eye hard, even if it threatens the macula (see the anti-VEGF section below, first).

If the patient already has a fairly full PRP, you need to pull out all the stops and squeeze in treatment anywhere you can—such patients need dead retina, and lots of it. You should aggressively try to fill in between spots, and also try to get out to the ora. This almost always involves fancier techniques, such as indirect laser or even cryotherapy, especially if the view is poor. If there is no view due to vitreous hemorrhage or cataract, the patient needs to be referred for whatever surgery is necessary to get to the retina and treat it. By the way, if a cataract is obscuring the view and preventing treatment, avoid just popping out the cataract and waiting for the eye heal before moving on to the laser. Cataract surgery can stimulate the new vessels go berserk, so get the PRP in quickly before everything falls apart.

If you don't have any way to get the PRP in at the time of cataract surgery, then try to do it shortly thereafter. Afraid to touch a post-op eye? First of all, if you think you will need to work on such an eye, put a stitch or two in the wound—you are dealing with problems that are way bigger than post-op astigmatism. If you are doing cataract surgery where they can't afford the equipment that allows small-incision phaco (for instance, if you are doing extracapsular surgery or even small-incision extracapsular surgery), remember that you can use a 90-D lens for a "no touch" PRP as discussed in Chapter 16. This is also a good indication for using an indirect ophthalmoscope delivery system, if you have access to one, but you still may not be able to easily treat beyond the equator because one still has to push on the eye hard to treat out there.

Anti-Vascular Endothelial Growth Factor (Anti-VEGF) Agents for Anterior Segment Neovascularization.

Anterior segment neovascularization can be a great indication for intravitreal anti-VEGF therapy if you have access to it (and assuming any posterior proliferative disease is controlled—see Chapter 11 for details). Although aggressive laser is the mainstay of treatment—injections are transient but the laser is permanent—intravitreal treatment can slow down the disease, giving you time to treat the patient gradually. Anti-VEGF drugs can also help protect the macula if fast and furious laser is needed, and chronic intravitreal treatment may be the only way to save the eye if the patient already has maximal laser. The exact approach and timing of intravitreal treatment has yet to be determined in this setting, but more and more it is becoming first-line therapy (bevacizumab is the most commonly used agent).

Keep in touch with your friendly neighborhood retina specialist to learn the latest thoughts, and have a very low threshold for considering this treatment if it is an option. By the way, there is a growing literature about the use of intracameral bevacizumab for this problem.[3] If you feel uncomfortable poking holes in the eye in places where you do not routinely operate, you can look into this if you are interested.

References and Suggested Reading

1.   Browning DJ. Risk of missing angle neovascularization by omitting screening gonioscopy in patients with diabetes mellitus. Am J Ophthalmol 1991;112:212.

2.   Fernandez-Vigo J, Castro J, Macarro A. Diabetic iris neovascularization. Natural history and treatment. Acta Ophthalmol Scand 1997;75:89-93.
Blinder KJ, Friedman SM, Mames RN. Diabetic iris neovascularization. Am J Ophthalmol 1995;120:393-5.

3.   Chalam KV, Gupta SK, Grover S, Brar VS, Agarwal S. Intracameral Avastin dramatically resolves iris neovascularization and reverses neovascular glaucoma. Eur J Ophthalmol. 2008 Mar-Apr;18(2):255-62.

Gartner S, Henkind P. Neovascularization of the iris (rubeosis iridis). Surv Ophthalmol 1978;22:291-312.

Ino-ue M, Azumi A, Shirabe H, Yamamoto M. Iridopathy in eyes with proliferative diabetic retinopathy: detection of early stage of rubeosis iridis. Ophthalmologica 1998;212:15-8.

Teich SA, Walsh JB. A grading system for iris neovascularization. Prognostic implications for treatment. Ophthalmology 1981;88:1102-6.

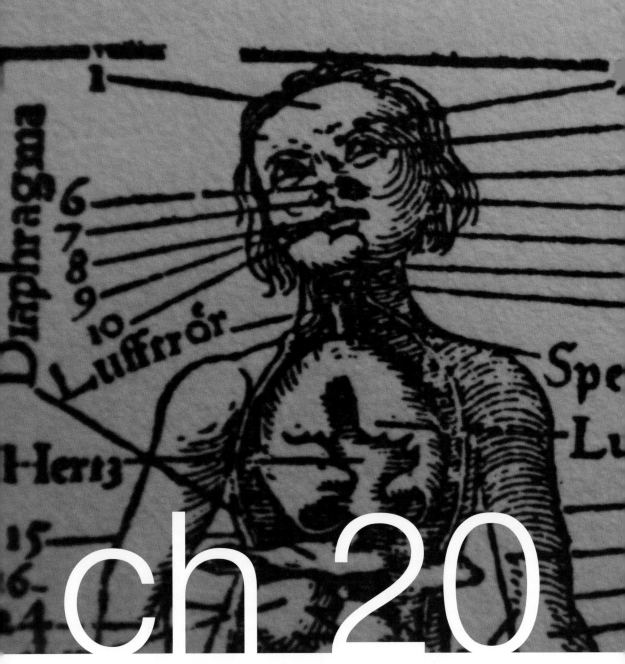

ch 20

The Most Useful Chapter in the Book
(But You Wouldn't Read It If It Had an Informative Title)

Don't blow off this chapter because you think you know it already. You can do the finest PRP in the world, yet you will be amazed at how you are largely wasting your time if your patient is noncompliant. The converse is also true. When you see how a set of eyes can improve when a patient gets religious about control, and how your treatments work way better in such patients, you will realize that it is definitely worth the time to rag on your patients about their systemic status.

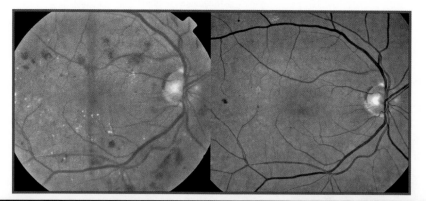

Figure 1. This patient had some mild grid laser to the center but, most importantly, she really began to take care of herself once she realized that the writing was on the wall. Note the almost total resolution of the multiple hemorrhages and the overall healthier appearance of the fundus after several years of better systemic control. No laser-slinger can do this by treating microaneurysms alone.

There are only a few risk factors that need to be covered. The most obvious one is glucose control, and the quickest way assess this is to ask the patient what their hemoglobin A1c is. Almost all patients will check their sugars periodically, and they may even remember some of their results (especially the best ones), but a sporadic sampling of glucose levels does not convey the overall level of control. In developed countries there is no reason why a patient should not be aware of their hemoglobin A1c level, although sometimes it helps if you call it the "three-month glucose test" if a patient does not recognize the test by name. Simply finding out whether they have heard of the test is useful—if they do not know what you are talking about, then you know you have a really big problem. Such a patient needs to be educated about the test and you need to express your concerns to their primary care physician. You can even order the test yourself to be sure it is done and to motivate both the patient and their doctor. Do not accept an answer like "My sugar is good." This isn't 1973.

Most patients will know the about the test, and even if they do not know their actual number, they can tell you whether their doctor was happy with the results. Knowing the actual number is best, though. A good number means that your treatment juju is strong. A bad number may completely change your ophthalmic management. What is a good number? A quick review may be in order…

Rapid Review of the Hemoglobin A1c Test

Glucose in blood sticks to all kinds of proteins like barnacles on a pier; the technical term for this is glycosylation. The higher the glucose level, the higher the amount of glycosylated proteins. Hemoglobin is one of these things to which glucose gets stuck. Red blood cells last two to three months, and because they do not manufacture fresh hemoglobin, measuring the fraction of hemoglobin that has been glycosylated offers an idea of the average glucose level over that time period. The test is basically a variation of the hemoglobin electrophoresis that one might do to evaluate for sickle cell disease, but one is looking for the hemoglobin fraction that has the glucose moiety, rather than hemoglobin S. The result is expressed as a percentage of the total hemoglobin. The translation of the A1c value into the corresponding glucose value varies with the testing method, and the actual result implies a range of values. For instance, a hemoglobin A1c of 6% implies a glucose value between 100-152. Table 1 shows the "average" glucose value that can be inferred from the hemoglobin A1c. Normal is less than 6%. Most diabetologists like to shoot for 7% or less. Seven to 8 is a gray zone—it is high but it may be the best that some patients can do. Eight or above is not good.

Table 1 / Hemoglobin A1c Values and Corresponding Average Glucose Level

Note that even the "good" value of 7% corresponds to a consistently elevated glucose.

(Data from: Nathan DM, et. al. Translating the A1C assay into estimated average glucose values. Diabetes Care. 2008 Aug;31(8):1473-8.)

A1c (%)	Mean Blood Sugar (mg/dl)
6	126
7	154
8	183
9	212
10	240
11	269
12	298

The risk of complications starts to go up almost asymptotically as the hemoglobin A1c increases. The classic paper on the subject is the Diabetes Control and Complications Trial (often just referred to as the DCCT).[1] Data from the study was used to create Figure 2, and this figure should be burned into your brain—it shows how bad control can undo the results produced by the laser. (Compare Figure 2 to the graphs in the chapters on the effects of laser on macular edema and proliferative disease. Your laser can change the linear slope of disease progression, but it can't completely overcome the skyward acceleration that occurs with poor control.) If you know a patient has bad systemic control, then your ophthalmic management may need to change.

> **If you have a lot of patients** that do not know their number, you can even buy or lease your own hemoglobin A1c machine in order to immediately get results. The test only requires a finger stick, and the machine does not require sophisticated training.

For instance, a patient with poor control should be checked more frequently than normal because they are very likely to progress faster. You may also need to be more aggressive about treatment decisions when patients have border-line ophthalmic disease. As an example, a patient with severe nonprolifera-tive retinopathy and good control may simply need to be watched, whereas a patient with the same level of retinopathy but with very poor control may need to be treated with an early PRP to stay out of trouble. Of greatest significance is the fact that a bad hemoglobin A1c means that you really have to take time to make sure the patient has appropriate expectations with any treatment that you do, whether it be laser, cataract surgery or whatever. Patients with poor control simply have a worse prognosis for everything, and they must understand that although your interventions will slow things down, the odds are they will tend to worsen, even with perfect treatment.

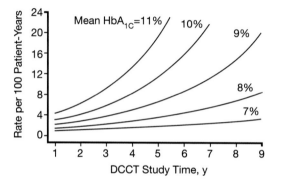

Figure 2. Rate of Retinopathy Progression Relative to Mean Hemoglobin A1c. (The relationship of glycemic exposure (HbA1c) to the risk of development and progres-sion of retinopathy in the Diabetes Control and Complications Trial. *Diabetes*. 1995;44:968-983.)

By the way—be careful how you harangue the patient about improving their control. Be sure to have them work with their internist before they start to do anything. The last thing you need is for the patient to bottom out their glu-cose on their own because you scared them so much.

Other Factors to Consider

There are other systemic factors that can play a role in progression of retinopa-thy. Four significant ones are hypertension, renal failure, lipid abnormalities and anemia. In fact, these factors can cause acute deterioration of a patient's retin-opathy in a far worse way than poor glucose control alone. For instance, it is not unusual to see patients who present with progressive renal failure and macular edema, only to have the edema resolve without laser as soon as the renal failure is treated.

Hypertension is particularly well studied—the sine qua non coming from the United Kingdom Prospective Diabetes Study Group.[2] Elevated blood pressure can be as important as glucose control—both in terms of contributing to chronic damage and causing acute problems in the setting of accelerated hyperten-sion. It makes sense to routinely check the blood pressure on diabetic patients, especially if it is not clear how good the patient is with their medical follow up. Yes, you might end up writing more letters, and you might actually have to check some blood pressures yourself, and you may even need to do general medical things like putting the patient in a room to calm down and then rechecking their blood pressure. It is worth it, though, because you will be surprised at the number of patients who are not as well controlled as they tell your technicians. It also helps to encourage patients to talk to their doctors about home blood pressure monitoring in the same way they monitor their glucose—automatic blood pressure cuffs are effective and cheap. By the way, current recommendations for blood pressure control in diabetics suggest that the goal should be to maintain pressures less than 130/80—the old "140/90" rule does not seem to be safe enough. Also, do not write off a high blood pressure as being due to "white coat syndrome." Such patients are more likely to get into trouble in the long run and should be monitored closely. [3]

Dyslipidemia also seems to accelerate the progression of retinopathy. Although there are, as yet, no large controlled studies looking at the effect of lipid control on retinopathy progression—such as there have been with glycemic control and hypertension—it is felt that lowering serum lipids is another important way to decrease the risk of vision loss for diabetic patients.[4] You will certainly see some patients with excessive amounts of hard exudates who will noticeably improve once their lipids are treated. (An example of exuberant hard exudate formation can be seen in Chapter 5.)

Diabetic nephropathy can also be associated with retinopathy progression.[5] This is particularly true if the patient has rapidly progressive renal failure, and this is always something to assess in a patient with very aggressive retinopathy. Remember that the converse also applies: By the time patients have retinopathy, they may also be developing renal disease. Make sure you remind the primary care physician to monitor renal function and look for microalbuminuria* in a patient who is beginning to get retinopathy. You should always include the patient's endocrinologist and nephrologist in your communications. Although it is easier (and cheaper) to just send a letter to the primary care physician, these medical subspecialists are in a good position to use the information you provide them in order to get the patient as tuned-up as possible.

Anemia also seems to play a role in retinopathy progression. Treating anemia in diabetes is known to have beneficial effects such as slowing progression of nephropathy, enhancing cognitive function and improving exercise capacity. Although there are no large randomized trials on this issue, it is felt that treatment of significant anemia may help slow retinopathy progression, especially if the

*Recall that the typical urine dipstick is not sensitive enough to detect the small amount of protein that can indicate the presence of early nephropathy. Special testing is required.

anemia is secondary to kidney disease.[6]

All of the above factors—glucose control, hypertension, renal failure, dyslipidemia and anemia—are important when it comes to both the patient's overall health and their response to your treatment. You should consider them inseparable when counseling patients and their doctors, and you should always stress the need to monitor all of them. Have your transcriptionist create a macro so you can easily throw in a comment about all of these in every letter you write. For instance:

The patient understands how important it is to work with their physician to optimize not only their glucose control, but also any element of hypertension, elevated cholesterol, early renal failure and anemia.

See how easy that was?

> **By the way,** if the patient improves thanks to the efforts of their medical doctors, you should definitely communicate this in your letters. It is a good feeling to snatch someone from the jaws of blindness, and most of the time we in ophthalmology get to take all the credit for doing this. In the setting of diabetes, however, nothing we do works very well if the patient is not systemically controlled. Taking the time to thank everyone for their help and to let them know they aided in avoiding blindness will certainly juice up their day. It may also encourage them to do the same thing for all their other patients, and because the best treatment for retinopathy is to avoid it in the first place one can create a very nice ripple effect by providing the positive feedback.

Some More Factors

Smoking is a factor that one would assume to be a real problem when it comes to exacerbating retinopathy. However, there is not as strong an association as one would think. The literature goes back and forth on the issue, and it is therefore not fully justified to include smoking with the above pantheon of clear-cut risk factors.[7] However, smoking clearly worsens other problems, such as large-vessel disease and renal failure, and these in turn can exacerbate retinopathy. Besides, smoking can aggravate other ophthalmic problems such as cataracts and macular degeneration, so you should feel free to nag patients about their smoking, whether they have diabetes or not. The American Academy of Ophthalmology makes a nice handout on the subject of smoking and its effects on the eye. Unfortunately, large corporations have worked very hard to make it very difficult to stop smoking, so it is not clear how much success you may have with this one. Sometimes, though, patients will be more worried about their eyes than lung cancer or emphysema, and by taking the time to warn them about smoking on the basis of your retinal exam you may get more mileage than their general medical doctors.

Additional factors that may play a role in retinopathy progression include obstructive sleep apnea, obesity, and physical inactivity.[8] Perhaps the strongest risk factor is duration of the disease, but this is not particularly modifiable without time travel. Finally, don't forget the potential effect of pregnancy on retinopathy (which can be so significant that it gets Chapter 23 all to itself).

Even More Factors to Consider

It would be great if this chapter could stop with that last paragraph, but there are some subtle nuances to consider when addressing issues of systemic control. Here they are:

Rapid Institution of Tight Control in Patients Who Have Been Poorly Controlled

The rapid institution of tight control can result in temporary worsening of diabetic retinopathy in some patients. This effect was best demonstrated in the DCCT, wherein motivated study patients were treated very aggressively and brought under control very quickly. The problem, if it occurs, tends to be transient and the long-term benefits of good control by far outweigh any temporary problems. It is more likely to occur in patients who have a history of very poor control and active retinopathy, and it has therefore been suggested that such patients should be brought under control slowly. In the real world, patients who have had poor control are usually incapable of improving things as rapidly as patients in the study, so this potential problem is usually not an issue. Still, you need to be aware of this possibility and watch for it in the appropriate setting.

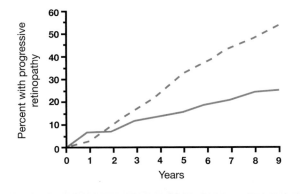

Figure 3. The effect of intensive control on progression of retinopathy. You can see the initial blip in the progression of retinopathy with rapid initiation of intensive control in the setting of this study. Note that even if this occurs there is a huge long-term benefit from maintaining good control. (Data from The Diabetes Control and Complications Trial Research Group, N Engl J Med 1993; 329:977. Courtesy of Uptodate.com)

If you do think you have a patient who has this problem, you have to be very careful about how you discuss it. First of all, it is never clear in a particular patient whether worsening is due to this phenomenon or whether it is just their natural history given their prior poor control. Second, you have to carefully explain that the long-term benefits of good control always trump any temporary short-term changes, because patients may mistakenly think that good control is now their enemy.

Caveats:

There are two specific situations in which the rapid institution of tight control can influence your ophthalmic management:

1. Pregnant diabetics have to be rapidly controlled to protect the fetus, and this phenomenon may be part of the reason why retinopathy can progress during pregnancy. See Chapter 23.
2. There is a paper suggesting that rapid institution of tight control may be especially problematic if it is done around the time of cataract surgery. See Chapter 24.

Lack of Immediate Gratification with Institution of Good Control

Although the preceding section discussed the transient effect of rapidly instituting tight control, a far more common problem from the standpoint of the patient is that once they actually manage to improve their control, they are almost never rewarded with total reversal of their diabetic complications.

This is the usual scenario: Around the time that you need to start treating them they also begin to get other systemic complications. They finally understand how important it is to control the risk factors discussed in this chapter, and for the first time in years they start to take better care of themselves. Unfortunately, there is a certain inertia to diabetic complications and things tend to worsen in spite of their new control. They can easily draw the incorrect conclusion that it does not make any difference whether they maintain good control because they keep getting worse no matter how they live.

You have to discuss this carefully. If you quickly say, "You still have to pay for all your bad control in the past," what your patient may think is, "I have been trying my best and it sounds like I am going to get worse no matter what, so I might as well eat whatever I want."

Instead, you should point out that they are dealing with damage that began years ago, and that they cannot make this old damage suddenly disappear with good control. They need to understand that their eye disease is like a moving freight train: It takes a while to bring things to a halt. Fortunately, it always pays off to have better control—but it just takes a while for the patient to appreciate it. As you treat diabetics over time, you will have the opportunity to see patients who persevere with excellent control and actually reverse the level of their disease. Such experiences will make you a much better advocate for the importance of good control, because you *will* believe.

Even More Complicated Issues

Warning: Touchy-feely stuff coming up. Just shut up and read it.

As you review the importance of control, there may be certain patients who become overwhelmed with feelings of guilt about past indiscretions, i.e., they are going blind and it is totally their own fault. (Or they are made to feel this way by especially malignant family dynamics.) You do want them to be inspired to do better, but be aware that this type of guilt can make some patients so depressed that they are incapable of caring for themselves properly—especially if they are now afraid that they are going blind, too.

And it doesn't stop there…

Remember that, for some patients, the fact that you are treating them—or even just telling them that they have background retinopathy—may force them to face something they have been denying up until now: that diabetes will make the rest of their life very different from everyone else's. It could be that for the first time they have to confront their fears of ending up blind, amputated and dead at an early age. This is a *huge* issue to drop into someone's life, and you can totally miss the impact of this if you blast through the office visit in order to get on to the next patient. You can end up being utterly clueless about their inner life, and this is not a good way to be.

Try to listen beyond their questions and comments for signs of anxiety or depression. Don't hesitate to ask about these issues, or about symptoms of depression, and to inform the patient's other doctors if you are worried. It is possible that a few carefully chosen words about how diabetic complications are *not* inevitable may really ease their pain. The bulk of this book is about making sure that patients have appropriate expectations about our treatments. However, if you think your patient is mentally nosediving, you definitely want to make it clear that although there are never any guarantees it is rare for someone to go hopelessly blind from diabetes if they take care of themselves and are compliant with follow up (and they don't have horrible retinopathy).

There is a sense of balance to be struck here, as usual. If they are leaving Doritos crumbs in your laser room while they brag that their hemoglobin A1c of 10 is way better than it used to be, then you should throw the book at 'em. But if they are depressed and guilty, give them some reassurance—and get them help.

There is a reason why you are doing this work and not some laser robot that could do a better job of treating the retina than any of us anyway. Ophthalmologists tend to be spared the sturm and drang of mental health issues, but diabetics are more likely to be depressed and you can be far more helpful to your patients if you remain sensitive to this.

Diabetics often have another source of stress that may require your attention: problems at work caused by fluctuating vision. They may have transient difficulties, for instance with a vitreous hemorrhage, or they may have more chronic problems such as trouble with lighting or with using a computer. You may need to call or write to their employer to explain any special needs to help them keep their job. You may need to educate them about any vocational rehabilitation services that may be available. Of course, if there is too much fuss they can get fired—nothing is simple. It gets even more complicated for some patients because at times their vision may be bad enough to keep them from working but not bad enough to qualify for disability. This can put a tremendous amount of financial stress on the patient and their family. Finally, remember that if they can't work they will likely be unable to afford insurance, and this can literally be a matter of life and death for a diabetic. All of this means that you need to be sensitive to any employment-related issues and be ready to help in any way you can.

Summing Up

Everything in this chapter sounds like it could be a lot of work, and it seems to go way beyond the call of duty for the average ophtho-mechanic. It doesn't take more than a few moments, though, to ask about the various risk factors and listen for any indications that that patient may be getting frustrated or dangerously depressed about some of this. It is crucial to recognize that treating diabetic retinopathy involves acknowledging that the patient exists in a matrix far more complex than what you see in the retina or on your OCT. The matrix includes things like their socioeconomic status, their degree of sophistication and their emotional state, as well as whether they have hard exudates within 500 microns of the fovea. If all of these issues are not addressed it is impossible to get the best results possible with your treatments.

One More Thing…Diplomacy in Action…Is it the doctor or the patient?

As you delve into a patient's medical care you need to get some idea about how aggressive their medical doctor is when it comes to controlling all of their risk factors. Sometimes the patient will tell you that their doctor doesn't do very much for them. If this happens, try to avoid riding any excessively high horses until you have learned all the facts. Although righteous indignation is a fun emotion in Hollywood epics about the struggle between good and evil, it should not be your default response to a patient who complains that their doctor does not seem to care about their diabetes. It is far more likely that the patient is poorly motivated, and their otherwise-busy healthcare providers have recognized this and therefore do not pour a lot of effort into the patient's management. A high-handed letter from the ophthalmologist demanding to know why no one has checked the HbA1c and insisting that everything be fixed straight away will not accomplish much, especially if the medical team has, in fact, been trying to do this for years. It is best to start slowly by communicating your findings and concerns, and then watching for the results. A phone call to the patient's doctor may also be invaluable to get the full story—it is all too easy for a patient to blame a doctor rather than blame themselves. If, after all this, the patient still isn't getting the kind of care you think they need then you can begin to assume there is a problem with the caregivers.

It could be that their health care providers may be too busy, poorly motivated, or just not up to speed on the best management. A recent study looking at quality of care for adult diabetics showed that *only 7.3%* attained recommended goals of an HbA1c level less than 7%, a blood pressure less than 130/80 mm Hg, and a total cholesterol level less than 200 mg/dL. In fact, two in five had poor LDL cholesterol control, one in three had poor blood pressure control, and one in five had a hemoglobin A1c that was over 9%.[9]

You may need to be the one that nudges both the patient and their doctor in the right direction—and you may even need to start by being the one that checks the blood pressure and gets all the various tests such as hemoglobin A1c and renal function studies. Another approach would be to suggest to the patient that they discuss with their doctor the option of getting an endocrinology consult if they are having problems getting their glucose under control. If you really feel that no progress is being made, you may even have to make a referral to a diabetologist on your own.

All this may involve treading a fine line between being helpful and ticking off your medical colleagues—but ultimately the best interest of the patient has to prevail. Knowing your medical community, and knowing each doctor's abilities, can be helpful here. Whatever you do, don't abrogate your role in the patient's care by whining that "it's someone else's job." It has to be your job because your outcomes depend on it.

Look at it this way: Systemic control is fundamental to the success of your ophthalmic interventions in the same way that implanting the proper IOL is important to your surgical results. You would never let a patient haphazardly pull their own IOL out of the pile. You should consider the treatment of diabetic retinopathy in the same way—never allow a patient to screw up your fine work with poor control if there is anything at all you can do to help it.

One last blue box thought: If patients actually listen to you and their other doctors and improve their glucose control, recognize that a visit to your office may now represent a real threat to their health. If you get backed up and they have to wait a long time to be seen they can easily become hypoglycemic. Always keep some orange juice or some other form of glucose around the office so that patients can be readily treated if this happens.

References and Recomended Reading

1.	The effect of intensive treatment of diabetes on the development and progression of long-term complications in insulin-dependent diabetes mellitus. The Diabetes Control and Complications Trial Research Group. N Engl J Med 1993;329:977-86.
2.	Tight blood pressure control and risk of macrovascular and microvascular complications in type 2 diabetes: UKPDS 38. UK Prospective Diabetes Study Group. BMJ 1998;317:703-13.
3.	Arauz-Pacheco C, Parrott MA, Raskin P. The treatment of hypertension in adult patients with diabetes. Diabetes Care 2002;25:134-47.
4.	Leiter LA. The prevention of diabetic microvascular complications of diabetes: is there a role for lipid lowering? Diabetes Res Clin Pract 2005;68 Suppl 2:S3-14.
5.	Cruickshanks KJ, Ritter LL, Klein R, Moss SE. The association of microalbuminuria with diabetic retinopathy. The Wisconsin Epidemiologic Study of Diabetic Retinopathy. Ophthalmology 1993;100:862-7.
6.	Sinclair SH, Malamut R, Delvecchio C, Li W. Diabetic retinopathy: treating systemic conditions aggressively can save sight. Cleve Clin J Med 2005;72:447-54.
7.	Aiello LP, Cahill MT, Wong JS. Systemic considerations in the management of diabetic retinopathy. Am J Ophthalmol 2001;132:760-76.
8.	Mohamed Q, Gillies MC, Wong TY. Management of diabetic retinopathy: a systematic review. JAMA 2007;298:902-16.
9.	Saydah SH, Fradkin J, Cowie CC. Poor control of risk factors for vascular disease among adults with previously diagnosed diabetes. JAMA 2004;291:335-42.

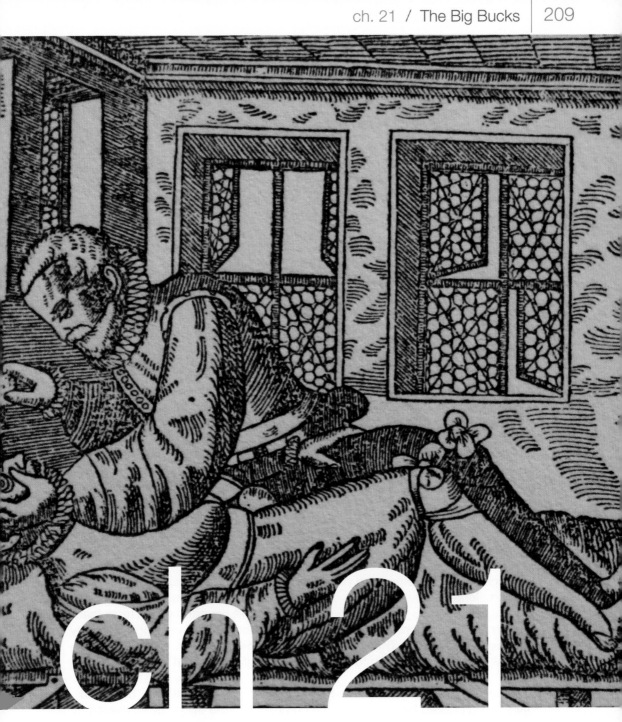

ch 21

The Big Bucks

THE BIG BUCKS

Unless you are reading this as you lug your laser to the nearest free clinic, it is likely that you will be involved in some sort of economic transaction when you treat a patient. If you are in a developed country that has universal health coverage, you can stop reading this right now because this section does not apply to you. If you are in a developing country, then you do need to worry about this stuff because there are insufficient healthcare resources available to cover the population. There are some suggestions about what to do at the end of this chapter (and at the end of Chapter 6).

If you are living in America, reportedly the richest country on earth, you really need to read this because you will inevitably have patients with no way to afford their medical care. Go figure.

At the beginning of your career there is a tendency to focus on the difficult task of being the best doctor you can be and it is therefore easy to be unaware of the socioeconomic ramifications of what you are doing. There is an inclination to surrender your control in this area to whatever large bureaucratic structure you happen to be a part of—this way some other functionary has to fuss with droll matters like billing and collections while you concentrate on the noble task of being a physician. Try not to think like this if you can help it; patients can make extremely bad decisions in this situation. Here's how:

Many of your diabetic patients will not have insurance. Being diabetic, it is hard to get a job with good insurance, and it is essentially impossible to purchase individual insurance. Many diabetics learn to survive without insurance by paying for their medical care on an intermittent basis and/or with the help of charity clinics. This is not ideal, and this approach usually breaks down when they start to develop complications and need more expensive care (which is where you come in).

Imagine you are an otherwise young and healthy diabetic, but now you are getting proliferative disease. Some doctor is telling you that even though you don't have any symptoms you need to sit down and get pounded with a laser that will hurt, maybe blur up your side vision, and probably not do anything to actually improve how you see. Then you go talk to the billing person, and they tell you that all of this bliss is going to cost thousands of dollars that you don't have.

The point is that a physician can be totally caring and empathetic, but a relatively disinterested bean counter can completely undo things by inadvertently making patients visualize eating cat food in order to pay for something that they don't want to do anyway. Some of these patients will walk away and not be treated. They will then return in one to two years with severe proliferative disease and tractional detachments that may not be fixable. It turns out that this works out well for the accounts receivable department, because now the patient is blind and they are at least eligible for Medicaid—some blood can finally be squeezed out of their particular turnip. You—and the Great Ophthalmologic Court in the Sky judging our actions—should be somewhat less than sanguine about how the system allows this to happen.

This scenario simply should not occur, but it does, due to the nature of human beings and the nature of our healthcare system. You may well be in a position to stop this from happening, given that only you know how desperately such a patient needs treatment. If you try just to be a good doctor—without considering the patient's worries about money—you may be failing at your goal.

Take a moment to look at the patient's chart to see if they have insurance. Do a little bit of ACLU-proscribed profiling. If you think money might be an issue, then you should consider bringing it up. And you need to do it *carefully*. Most patients, especially patients in this situation, will immediately assume that any time a doctor brings up money, it means that the doctor is simply performing a wallet biopsy prior to putting on the big squeeze. It behooves you to quickly explain why you are exploring this issue. Remind them that they desperately need the treatment to avoid blindness, and you want to make sure that they get treated properly whether they can pay or not.

The alternatives available to you depend on how much control you have over your billing. It is likely that if you are reading this book you are in training or just starting your career and you may be unable to control how patients are billed. If cost is an issue for the patient you should try to take a moment to explain to the billing person the severity of the situation, making sure they know to go as easy as possible on the patient. (Depending on the situation, one can even consider doing the laser without circling the laser code on the billing sheet. This could be dangerous ground—for instance, Medicare considers doing a procedure without billing for it to be fraud, no matter how noble the cause. Still, if you are trying to keep a patient from going blind you need to at least think about all your options. Hopefully someone somewhere will realize how utterly illogical all of this is and the system will be fixed.)

If you have more control over your situation, you can tell the patient they can set up some sort of payment plan, or you can even bargain over the price if you are so inclined. Probably the simplest thing is to offer to do the treatment gratis. This eliminates any financial stress, and offering to do something regardless of payment is a very powerful way to demonstrate to a patient the importance of the treatment. You may actually find that such a patient will remain quite devoted to you, and you may find that the whole process is rather rewarding on a number of warm and fuzzy levels that are beyond the scope of this book.

If such an approach does not fit into your world view, consider a more cynical argument for this policy: Recognize that if you can keep them functioning in society, they will certainly think of you when they do eventually get insurance and may need elective procedures. They will also speak very highly of you to all of their friends, family, and other doctors and, yes, there may be a risk of inundating your office with their equally uninsured acquaintances—but it is far more likely that the long-term goodwill you acquire in the community is going to transcend any short-term irregularities in your cash flow. On an even grander note, it is a little-known fact that Dante's Inferno mentions that there is a spot reserved for American ophthalmologists somewhere in the Fourth Circle of Hell. (Dante said it had something to do with taking drug company swag.) It is likely that

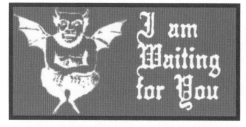

doing the right thing for patients like this will get you a few weekends of vacation up in Purgatory. Everybody wins.

The bottom line on the bottom line is that it is hard enough to convince diabetics to show up for evaluation and treatment without adding financial impediments. Although it is technically not part of your job description, try to be aware of economic hurdles that your patients may be facing. Otherwise, you might as well stop practicing medicine until someone figures out a way to unscrew eyeballs, put them in Petri dishes, and treat them on an assembly line. You can pick whatever reason you want—just try not to let the billing department define your patient's treatment options.

This chapter really applies only to doctors in the USA. As mentioned at the beginning of this section, doctors in developing countries have a related problem, and it has to do with the fact that there are likely tons of patients in need of help, but there are no resources to help with paying for their care.

If you are in this situation, it turns out that there are a lot of organizations out there that are interested in helping—you just have to start making the effort to contact them. It is very likely that someone, somewhere has already faced the problems you are having, and has figured out a way to deal with it—and often quite successfully. The world is full of places that have skillfully combined capitalism and altruism to create very effective, self-sustaining programs that reward both the population and the doctors who take the time to go beyond their borders and ask for help. You have to be prepared to hear "no" many times, though, for every "yes"—but the yeses will add up if you are persistent.

The end of Chapter 6 lists some resources to give you a start…

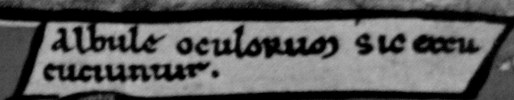

albule oculorum sic eueu
euciuntur.

ch 22
Diabetic Papillopathy

Or Non-Arteritic Ischemic Optic Neuropathy
That Happens to Occur in Diabetics.

Or Whatever...

This is an entity that does not quite fit into the categories of non-proliferative or proliferative disease. It is traditionally considered a relatively mild problem, but on occasion, it can be a real pain because it may create both a diagnostic and therapeutic challenge. It can also be easy to miss, especially if the patient has a lot of widespread macular edema that masks subtle swelling on the temporal aspect of the optic nerve. You do not want to miss it, though, because it adds a potential wild card to the patient's visual prognosis, and it is far better to recognize the problem and educate the patient than to be surprised. This is particularly true if a patient has vision loss due to papillopathy at some point after a laser; it is hard to retroactively convince the patient that the laser did not cause the problem.

Diabetic papillopathy was originally described in juvenile (Type 1) diabetic patients, but since then it has been described in older, Type 2 patients as well. The problem is most likely related to capillary damage that results in chronic ischemia and secondary nerve swelling, which, for reasons known only to the gods of diabetes, does not tip the nerve into full-blown ischemic optic neuropathy (usually). Perhaps the nerve doesn't lapse into full-fledged visual loss because the vascular system just isn't that bad—something which may go along with it occurring in younger patients. The possibility of some other form of metabolic insufficiency in the optic disc—for example, tissue anoxia due to poor glucose utilization or build-up of toxic substances related to diabetes—has also been entertained.

Pundits spend a great deal of time arguing about whether this entity is truly different from non-arteritic anterior ischemic optic neuropathy (NAION), or whether it is just an extremely benign form of NAION. It really does not make any difference, because you will still be biting your fingernails and hoping that it just goes away without causing any problems. Fortunately, this is indeed what happens to most patients, which is a good thing given the utter lack of proven treatments.

Many patients have no symptoms, and the problem is then identified incidentally upon clinical examination. Patients who do have symptoms tend to have non-specific blurring that is mild and intermittent, but patients with more severe disease may have marked visual changes. The vision tends to be only mildly affected, with most patients having better than 20/50 vision initially. There is usually little, if any, afferent pupillary defect unless there is significant and asymmetric loss of visual function—although if there is significant visual loss as evidenced by a large afferent papillary defect and visual field loss, one would tend not to diagnose diabetic papillopathy but rather NAION. The disc edema tends to be mild to moderate, with dilated capillaries in the superficial layers of the nerve, and often some splinter hemorrhages. The cup-to-disc ratio, if it can be evaluated, tends to be small and crowding at the nerve may play a part in this disease, not unlike typical non-arteritic ischemic optic neuropathy. Occasionally, patients may have little or no associated diabetic retinopathy, but most patients will have some degree of background diabetic retinopathy which may vary from mild disease to significant macular edema and even proliferative disease. About half of the time the disease is bilateral, although not always simultaneously.

An angiogram can be very helpful, because it will light up the nerve in a very characteristic way, which may help you avoid the embarrassment of missing the diagnosis in subtle cases. There are usually very obvious swollen vessels within the nerve substance that cause late staining that can mimic the appearance of proliferative disease if you don't look carefully. Studying the nerve, though, shows that the staining is limited to the nerve and that there are no overlying new vessels causing the leakage.

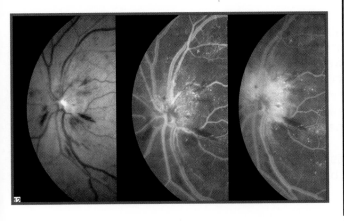

Figure 1. Diabetic papillopathy. The red free photo shows swelling of the nerve fiber layer with loss of the disc margins. There are also nerve fiber layer hemorrhages. The early phase of the angiogram shows typical dilated vessels and the late phase shows staining within the substance of the nerve which nicely backlights the overlying nerve fiber layer hemorrhages.

The visual field usually demonstrates enlargement of the physiologic blind spot, even in asymptomatic patients, although more pronounced constriction or altitudinal changes occur in more severe disease (and again, some would just call this type of vision loss NAION). Overall, the visual prognosis is relatively good, with most patients ending up 20/50 or better unless other aspects of their diabetic retinopathy intervene. There is a subset, perhaps 5 to 15%, who end up with significantly worse vision, and this may be the result of progression to frank NAION or, at times, from associated macular edema (which can be very treatable, so don't forget to look for it while you stare at the nerve). As a general rule, the patients who are younger and who present with minimal symptoms and findings tend to do best. Older patients with long-standing systemic vascular disease are more likely to end up with poor vision, especially if they present with worse disease.

A notable thing about this entity is that it takes many months for the edema to resolve, which is different from the relatively rapid resolution that occurs with ischemic optic neuropathy. The swelling usually begins to diminish by three to six months, although some patients have persistent swelling for a year or so. There is usually not a lot of pallor in the involved nerve once the swelling re-solves unless there has been significant nerve fiber damage. There are some patients, however, for whom the presence of diabetic papillopathy heralds the onset of more progressive traditional problems, such as proliferative disease or worsening macular edema. As a result, even if the nerve swelling subsides nicely patients with this entity need continued close monitoring.

Aspects of Diabetic Papillopathy That Can Be Problematic...

Although diabetic papillopathy is fairly benign most of the time, it has the potential to make trouble for two reasons: (1) the differential diagnosis can be a morass, and (2) it can be an unpredictable time bomb in terms of visual acuity.

DIFFERENTIAL DIAGNOSIS Issues

Unfortunately, when it comes to the differential diagnosis, there is nothing about the clinical exam that can definitively distinguish diabetic papillopathy from more ominous causes of optic nerve swelling. Most authors suggest that the diagnosis of diabetic papillopathy can be made if the patient is in the appropriate demographic and the vision and visual field are relatively reserved. This sounds reasonable, but one is still stuck with a patient who has a swollen optic nerve and, as a result, diabetic papillopathy is really a diagnosis of exclusion.

Although the differential diagnosis of optic nerve swelling is legion, here are some things to at least consider before simply deciding a patient has diabetic papillopathy:

A mild central retinal vein occlusion can have associated disc edema, especially in younger patients. The associated venous tortuosity and engorgement, and characteristic hemorrhages, should suggest venous occlusive disease. Optic neuritis can also cause disc swelling, but there are usually more pronounced effects on vision, and patients generally have the typical pain on movement associated with this entity.

Inflammatory or infectious disc swelling usually has an associated cellular infiltrate of the retina and/or vitreous, which suggests something more than plain old diabetic papillopathy. Examples include disc swelling in association with anterior or intermediate uveitis, or infectious causes such as cat-scratch disease or toxoplasmosis. Other more obscure entities such as orbital tumors, congenital abnormalities, or infiltrative lesions may need to be considered in the appropriate setting, but this all begins to get into very different clinical presentations. If you are really worried about this kind of stuff, you need to be reading a textbook with the word "neuro" in the title.

Finally, there are occasional patients who may develop vitreous traction inserting on the nerve, and this can simulate the swelling caused by diabetic papillopathy. It is important to distinguish traction from papillopathy, though, because traction on the nerve can sometimes benefit from vitrectomy in order to avoid visual field loss (see Chapter 18).

The real problem with patients with unilateral disease is deciding whether they have ischemic optic neuropathy, which, in turn, is all about deciding whether they need an evaluation for giant cell arteritis. The best way to tell diabetic papillopathy from either arteritic or non-arteritic ischemic optic neuropathy is simply observation over time. Diabetic papillopathy usually resolves with little sequelae, unlike ischemic optic neuropathy, which usually leaves more pronounced pallor of the nerve and permanent visual field loss. Also, as mentioned, the swelling caused by diabetic papillopathy may last much longer than that caused by ischemic optic neuropathy. Unfortunately, once the specter of giant cell arteritis is raised, the concept of "observation over time" becomes an unaffordable luxury—waiting to see if the fellow eye goes irreversibly blind is no way to make a diagnosis.

For younger patients with presumed diabetic papillopathy and minimal visual changes, this is much less of an issue and observation is warranted (assuming you have ruled out the entities mentioned above). For older diabetics, you are obligated to perform an evaluation for temporal arteritis—especially if there is significant loss of function. This becomes even more problematic because the usual tests (erythrocyte sedimentation rate and C-reactive protein) tend to be a bit abnormal in older diabetic patients, and you may be forced to consider invasive maneuvers such as temporal artery biopsies and prednisone treatment. The perils of missing a diagnosis of giant cell arteritis are great, but so are the risks of putting an elderly diabetic on prednisone. Whichever way you go, please make sure you have documented your rationale, and strongly consider obtaining other opinions to support your gut feelings, especially if you decide the patient simply has diabetic papillopathy and you are going to observe them. (A full discussion regarding the diagnosis of temporal arteritis is beyond the scope of this book—you know where to look.)

Making the diagnosis of diabetic papillopathy becomes problematic for a different reason if the patient presents with bilateral disease. One then needs to consider increased intracranial pressure as well as all the other causes of disc swelling. It is very risky to simply attribute bilateral disc swelling to diabetic papillopathy because of the rather grave consequences for the patient if you happen to be wrong. Also, remember that if you decide to forego a neurologic evaluation, those swollen nerves will be staring you down for many months to come; although an MRI and LP are not without risk and cost, it is usually better to get the more worrisome aspects of the differential diagnosis out of the way first.

There may be times when you may feel fairly certain that a patient has diabetic papillopathy and not bilateral papilledema from an intracranial process. An example would be a younger patient with no symptoms of elevated intracranial pressure and no reason in their medical history or general exam to indicate that they are predisposed to developing increased intracranial pressure. In this situation, some feel that a spinal tap can be deferred. This begins to resemble the kind of thing that neuro-ophthalmologists are clearly best at; you should consider getting another opinion before you do nothing but observe the patient.

> **Also, never forget** that one of the most important things to do with bilateral swollen nerves is to dust off your blood pressure cuff and check for severe hypertension. One would want to be the first in line to diagnose this problem and not wait for the ER to make the diagnosis two days later.

If you have easy access to the various ophthalmic specialties (i.e., if you are in training at a program where you can actually talk to the staff), you can get a sense for just how much variability there can be when it comes to making this diagnosis. If you show a case that looks like diabetic papillopathy to a retina specialist, they will probably feel comfortable with simple observation, but if you show the same case to a neuro-ophthalmologist, you will likely be spending more time ruling out giant cell arteritis and/or elevated intracranial pressure. As a general rule, the neuro-ophthalmologist wins and you should consider diabetic papillopathy a diagnosis of last resort.

As an aside: Don't ever succumb to the illusory comfort that you are off the hook if you can get a retina specialist to commit to the easy diagnosis of diabetic papillopathy—especially if you are still worried about something else in your heart of hearts. Retina specialists may not know what they don't know when it comes to optic nerves, so just do what you think is the right thing.

A final point in the differential is that, sometimes, the dilated capillaries seen on the nerve with this entity can simulate neovascularization of the disc. In general, the vascular changes associated with papillopathy tend to be more radially oriented and are within the substance of the disc, whereas true neovascularization forms an irregular network above the surface of the disc. Also, true neovascularization tends to leak more on a fluorescein angiogram. However, because this entity can occasionally evolve into frank neovascularization you cannot just ignore the appearance of the vessels once you have decided the patient has diabetic papillopathy; instead, you need to watch them carefully to make sure that they do not sprout high-risk proliferative disease.

VISUAL ACUITY and Treatment Issues

OK. Having worked through the above diagnostic process, let's assume the patient actually has diabetic papillopathy. Fortunately, most patients end up doing well, but there are occasional patients who may develop severe vision loss, and this may occur at any point in time. It is particularly frustrating if it occurs around the time you have performed a laser to treat their macular edema or proliferative disease, because the patient will think their vision loss is your fault. Even if the patient does not have marked worsening of their vision, diabetic papillopathy can still limit visual recovery if patients have been treated for more reversible problems, such as cataracts or a vitreous hemorrhage. Finally, they need to know there is a chance this could evolve into high-risk neovascularization, bringing with it all the joys of panretinal photocoagulation. In essence, you have to be able to recognize this entity and, once it is recognized, you have to spend some time educating the patient about the potential problems it can cause—even if most patients do fine.

In terms of treatment, there is no proven approach. Like any other diabetic manifestation, the patient should be urged to control all of the usual vascular risk factors, as outlined in Chapter 20. Of course, the fact that there are no proven treatments means that, inevitably, you will find someone who is willing to inject something into the eye. As of this writing there is no definitive study to guide therapy, but there are some case reports suggesting that steroids, and perhaps bevacizumab, can be helpful. If the patient has marked vision loss, it may be worth considering trying something. The patient really needs to understand the potential risks and know that such treatment is undertaken in desperation— without a lot of support from the literature (for instance, no one knows what might happen to an ischemic nerve if it is exposed to a pressure in the 40s from steroid-induced ocular hypertension).

Ultimately, diabetic papillopathy is an entity that spans other specialties, so on the next page are some additional references that serve to further explore the subject. Neither this list of references nor this chapter is exhaustive. If you have a patient with diabetic papillopathy, you may want to run the case by your friendly neighborhood neuro-ophthalmologist to be sure you have a handle on the latest approaches to this disease.

References and Suggested Reading

Lubow M, Makley TA. Pseudopapilledema of juvenile diabetes mellitus. Arch Ophthalmol 1971;85:417.

Barr CC, Glaser JS, Blankenship G. Acute disc swelling in juvenile diabetes: clinical profile and natural history of 12 cases. Arch Ophthalmol 1980;98:2185.

Regillo CD, Brown GC, Savino PJ, et al. Diabetic papillopathy. Patient characteristics and fundus findings. Arch Ophthalmol 1995;113:889-95.

Hayreh SS. Diabetic papillopathy and nonarteritic anterior ischemic optic neuropathy. Surv Ophthalmol 2002;47:600-2; author reply 602.

Bayraktar Z, Alacali N, Bayraktar S. Diabetic papillopathy in type II diabetic patients. Retina 2002;22:752-8.

Saito Y, Ueki N, Hamanaka N, Shiotani Y, Nakae K, Kiuchi Y. Transient optic disc edema by vitreous traction in a quiescent eye with proliferative diabetic retinopathy mimicking diabetic papillopathy. Retina 2005;25:83-4.

Mansour AM, El-Dairi MA, Shehab MA, Shahin HK, Shaaban JA, Antonios SR. Periocular corticosteroids in diabetic papillopathy. Eye 2005;19:45-51.

Al-Haddad CE, Jurdi FA, Bashshur ZF. Intravitreal triamcinolone acetonide for the management of diabetic papillopathy. Am J Ophthalmol 2004;137:1151-3.

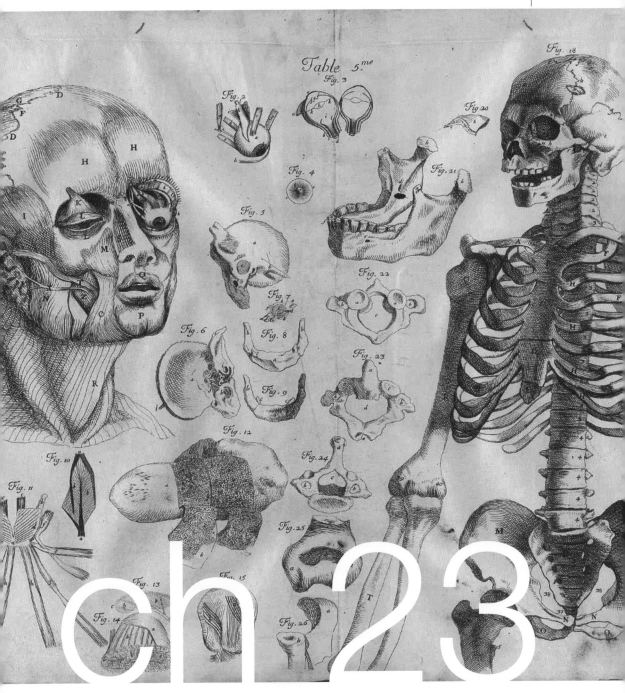

Proliferating While Proliferating:
Diabetic Retinopathy During Pregnancy

There is no question that diabetic retinopathy can worsen during pregnancy, but there is also a chance that this progression may spontaneously regress during the postpartum period. This means that treating retinopathy during pregnancy may require a little more flair than treating "standard" diabetics. There are four main variables that are important in determining a patient's risk for progression during pregnancy: (1) the degree of retinopathy present at the onset of pregnancy; (2) the duration of the patient's diabetes; (3) the level of control prior to the pregnancy; and (4) problems with hypertension during the pregnancy.

All patients should be examined during their first trimester. It makes sense to see patients with little or no retinopathy about every three months. If there is any significant retinopathy, then the intervals should be decreased, especially if the patient has a history of poor control that is suddenly improving in the setting of aggressive perinatal care. Patients presenting with moderate to severe disease may even need to be checked every month to monitor for progression.

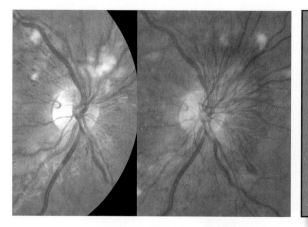

Figure 1. This patient went from no neovascularization on the left to the huge frond on the right over a two-month period in the second trimester. The irregular truncated capillaries and cotton wool spots around the nerve in the left photo suggest significant ischemia, and are a portent of real trouble. (Courtesy of William A. Argus, M.D.)

The most important exam, however, should occur well before a patient becomes pregnant. Ideally, a diabetic woman who is considering pregnancy should be informed about the status of her retinopathy and given some sort of idea about the potential risk that pregnancy poses to her vision. Fortunately, the risk is minimal in a conscientious patient with a history of good control, good follow up, and mild retinopathy.

It is also helpful if the patient can be evaluated by an endocrinologist (and nephrologist if necessary). These specialists can give the patient an idea of her systemic risk; for instance, pregnancy can accelerate nephropathy, which, in turn, is associated with an increased risk of fetal complications. If the patient is trying to decide whether to get pregnant and she is not being followed by such specialists, it may be incumbent on you to insist. If there is enough eye disease to get you involved in the decision, then the patient may need a specialist evaluation to get the best possible advice about other potential problems.

As an aside, there appears to be little or no risk of developing retinopathy in patients who are diagnosed with gestational diabetes and have no prior history of diabetes. Such patients are at increased risk for developing frank diabetes down the road, but routine eye exams during pregnancy are probably not necessary.[1] If there is any question about prior diabetes, though, an exam is warranted.

In terms of determining a given patient's risk of progression, the easiest thing to do from an ophthalmic standpoint is to categorize patients based on their pre-existing retinopathy. If there is no retinopathy present at the beginning of pregnancy, the odds are good that the patient will not develop any significant problems during the pregnancy. The patient still needs to be examined; there are studies suggesting it is possible for patients to develop problems such as macular edema or proliferative disease even if they have little or no pre-existing retinopathy at the start of pregnancy. Problems are, once again, more likely to develop in patients with a history of long-standing diabetes and poor control.

If the patient does have pre-existing retinopathy, it is hard to be very specific about her risk for progression because the literature is quite variable. Furthermore, many of the older papers had patients with poorer control compared to the average patient in the modern era, and bad control automatically worsens the prognosis. In general, the more severe the retinopathy, the more likely the progression.

One commonly quoted paper is the Diabetes in Early Pregnancy Study.[2] This showed that patients with no retinopathy, microaneurysms only, mild nonproliferative retinopathy, and moderate to severe nonproliferative retinopathy at baseline had progression of their retinopathy in 10.3, 21.1, 18.8, and 54.8% of patients, respectively. In this case, progression referred to worsening of their nonproliferative findings or the development of proliferative disease. (Significant progression of nonproliferative disease was defined as "two-step" progression. This means that the patient moved two steps along the scale of nonproliferative disease, i.e., from mild—past moderate—to severe disease.) The percentage of patients who developed proliferative disease was smaller, but still significant: Proliferative retinopathy developed in 6.3% of patients with mild disease at the onset of pregnancy, but it developed in as many as 29% of patients who began with moderate to severe retinopathy. It is likely that the risk is less presently. (This paper was published in 1995—a paper published six years later looking at patients with better control had an across-the-board progression rate to proliferative disease of only 2.2%.)[3]

All this data refers to patients with active disease. It turns out that if patients present with old proliferative disease that has been well controlled with previous treatment, they are much less likely to develop progression of their retinopathy during the pregnancy. There are, of course, no guarantees, but this demographic tends to be stable.

It is not clear why retinopathy progresses during pregnancy. It has been speculated to be caused by changes in cardiac output that "strain" the retinal circulation. There may also be hormonal influences. One likely factor is the effect of taking a patient whose control may have been marginal and rapidly improving their control. As mentioned in Chapter 20, the rapid institution of tight control can cause temporary worsening of retinopathy. This phenomenon doesn't make much difference in non-pregnant patients, because the long-term results clearly favor tight control and because most patients can't come under control quickly anyway. In the setting of pregnancy, however, there is a need to rapidly institute tight control in order to avoid complications such as congenital malformations and miscarriage. As a result, even if the rapid tightening of control is problematic for the retinas of pregnant patients, there really is no choice.

However, retinopathy progression is not entirely related to the institution of tight control. The fact that simply being pregnant contributes to progression is demonstrated by the observation that some patients who develop proliferative disease during pregnancy will experience spontaneous regression of the neovascularization in the postpartum period. This is not something to depend on, though, and it makes sense to treat proliferative disease during pregnancy rather than to watch it. For instance, if the patient is developing proliferative disease treatment should be considered even if she does not have high-risk features in order to avoid problems later in the pregnancy.

It is always bad if a pregnant patient somehow manages to present with brand new proliferative disease at her first visit. It is likely that such patients had very poor control, and they need to be treated immediately and followed closely. Another bad sign is if the patient has a history of treatment but begins to develop recurrent disease during pregnancy—one should aggressively fill in any pre-existing panretinal photocoagulation pattern to try and regain control of the disease. You may be interested to know that in the bad old days, the presence of aggressive retinopathy was considered an indication to abort the pregnancy—hopefully your laser can avoid such an outcome. On the other hand, if patients develop mild proliferative disease and have a history of good control, you can make a case for treating relatively lightly because, under these circumstances, you may simply need to get them through their pregnancy in hopes that the neovascular stimulus will resolve postpartum.

Basically, you need to assess each patient on a case-by-case basis—you can titrate the treatment depending on how aggressive their disease is and how precarious their medical situation is. If you are not sure how to proceed, a consultation is in order.

Whatever you do, all pregnant patients with proliferative disease require much more frequent monitoring than a non-pregnant patient—perhaps every two to four weeks—in order to be sure that the process is not worsening. You do not want such patients heading into the perinatal period with uncontrolled proliferative retinopathy. If they have any complications related to the delivery—or even if they are just figuring out how to get some sleep with a newborn at home—it may be weeks before you can get them into your office again.

One other thing: You have to be very careful about how you do your PRPs in this setting. Not only do you have to worry about all the usual stuff that can go wrong—like macular edema—but you also have to remember that for most people anything that causes eye pain can also induce vagal problems such as nausea. This is bad because pregnant women may be constantly on the verge of vomiting anyway, depending on where they are in their pregnancy. If you hit them with a lot of laser, and if they are particularly sensitive, you can throw them into an episode of diabetic ketoacidosis simply from pain and nausea and vomiting. This can happen even if you block them at the time of the laser—when your block wears off, they can still be miserable. This scenario is not a good thing for someone who is pregnant, and might cause more morbidity than the proliferative disease you are trying to treat. There is no magic solution here. You can use all the tricks in Chapter 15 on pain management. You can make sure the patient is working closely with her obstetrician and endocrinologist if she does have problems, and if she needs medication to treat any nausea those specialists can choose ones that are safe in pregnancy. You may also have to do several lasers using a small number of spots over many closely spaced visits, if necessary. Whatever it takes. Fortunately, this doesn't come up often, but it is a reminder of how much you need to be ready to customize your PRPs.

MACULAR EDEMA

Treating diabetic macular edema may also require a very different approach relative to treating non-pregnant patients. It is possible to be very conservative with these patients because treatment may not be necessary. One study suggested that as many as 88% of eyes that develop diabetic macular edema during pregnancy will undergo resolution of the edema without laser treatment.[4]

However, you need to consider treatment if the vision is markedly decreased or if there are areas of focal leakage that are allowing lipid to build up and threaten the fovea. It may also be necessary to treat patients who develop significant central thickening early in their pregnancy; it is not a good idea to leave the macula swollen for several months. As usual, there really is no definitive data that guides the approach in this situation, and you also have to look at the patient's systemic status and history of control. This is also a situation where one might consider referring for consideration of intravitreal triamcinolone, because it might buy these patients time to get to their delivery without putting permanent laser spots in their posterior pole.* This is not to say this is a totally ideal solution—endophthalmitis or glaucoma during pregnancy is not a good thing—but one should be flexible about how one approaches these patients. (Anti-vascular endothelial growth factor drugs are unlikely to be an option in this situation; it will be a long time before anyone can say how safe it is to use such drugs in someone whose uterus is filled with a growing baby.)

*Ophthalmic drug use in pregnancy could be the subject of an entire book itself. Although a fraction of a milliliter of triamcinolone into the vitreous is not likely to be a problem, always check with the obstetrician to cover yourself and *never* take a retina specialist's word on this. Next paragraph notwithstanding…

Fluorescein angiography? The decision to perform a fluorescein angiogram can be difficult in the setting of pregnancy. Although there is no report of teratogenicity associated with the use of fluorescein, almost everyone tries to avoid injecting things into pregnant women for all of the obvious reasons. It is felt that an angiogram is reasonably safe if the results would change the treatment approach in a patient facing the risk of blindness.[5] As a comprehensive ophthalmologist, it is unlikely that you would truly find yourself in this situation; any patient this complex should probably be referred. Besides, most of the worrisome changes that occur in a diabetic retina can be identified with a careful clinical examination alone. The risk of an angiogram probably outweighs any benefits in a typical situation—even if the risk is largely theoretical.

What about the actual delivery? There have been a few cases of vitreous hemorrhage reported during labor and delivery in patients with proliferative disease. However, there is some degree of risk to performing a cesarean section, and the general feeling is that, all things considered, it is probably safer to go ahead and have a vaginal delivery and avoid a cesarean section if the only reason for performing a cesarean section is the fear of a vitreous hemorrhage. We can always operate on a vitreous hemorrhage, and the morbidity associated with a cesarean section is more than that associated with a vitrectomy, especially for a diabetic patient. Be prepared for a phone call or two from the OB team, though. If it looks like this may be an issue, the patient might benefit from a referral well before the time of delivery.

Once the patient delivers, things tend to settle down from the standpoint of retinopathy progression. The exact schedule for follow up would depend on how much trouble occurred during the pregnancy. It might also be prudent to monitor patients who spontaneously improve postpartum in the event they regress in the first year after pregnancy, especially if they revert to poor control.

SUMMING UP

It is important to realize that the ramifications of treating retinopathy during pregnancy are significant; you are caring for at least two people. This section is really just an overview of what is a rather detailed literature. If there is any question about how to approach a given patient, you should explore this subject more deeply; the review by Brown and Sunness in particular is excellent.[6] You should also have a low threshold for asking for help—if a pregnant woman's eyes are in trouble the disease may behave very differently from typical retinopathy and the stakes are high.

References and Suggested Reading

1.   Puza SW, Malee MP. Utilization of routine ophthalmologic examinations in pregnant diabetic patients. J Matern Fetal Med 1996;5:7-10.

2.   Chew EY, Mills JL, Metzger BE, et al. Metabolic control and progression of retinopathy. The Diabetes in Early Pregnancy Study. National Institute of Child Health and Human Development Diabetes in Early Pregnancy Study. Diabetes Care 1995;18:631-7.

3.   Temple RC, Aldridge VA, Sampson MJ, Greenwood RH, Heyburn PJ, Glenn A. Impact of pregnancy on the progression of diabetic retinopathy in Type 1 diabetes. Diabet Med 2001;18:573-7.

4.   Sinclair SH, Nesler C, Foxman B, Nichols CW, Gabbe S. Macular edema and pregnancy in insulin-dependent diabetes. Am J Ophthalmol 1984;97:154-67.

5.   Sheth BP, Mieler WF. Ocular complications of pregnancy. Curr Opin Ophthalmol 2001;12:455-63.

6.   Brown, JC, Sunness JS. Pregnancy and Retinal Disease. In: Ryan SJ. Retina, 4th ed. Philadelphia: Elsevier Mosby, 2006:v.2, pp 1358-1363.

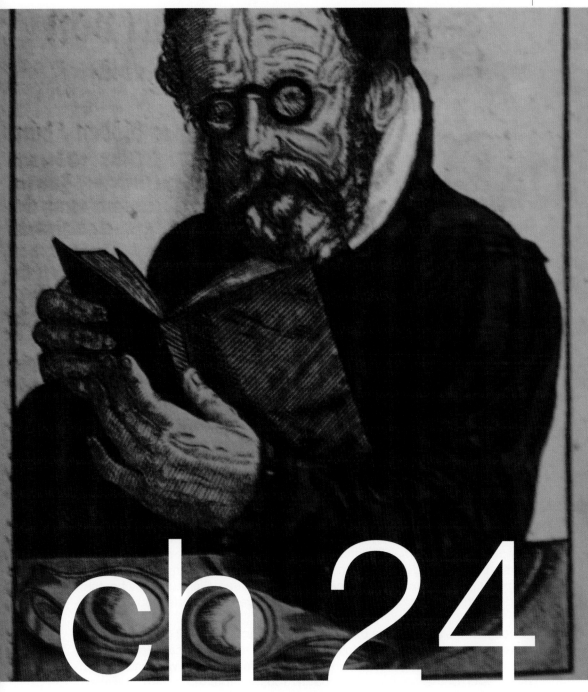

ch 24
Cataract Surgery & Diabetic Retinopathy

Not unlike the blind men who describe an elephant based on which part they are touching, there tends to be a big difference between how a retina specialist views cataract surgery in diabetics and how a cataract jockey views the issue. Retina people tend to be real worrywarts about this, and will be far more cautious about suggesting cataract surgery simply because of all the patients they have seen start with 20/40 glare cataracts and end up 20/200 from progression of their retinopathy after surgery. In the bad old days (a decade or two ago), it was not uncommon to hold off on cataract surgery until the vision was 20/200 or worse because, if things went south, the patient would at least have a fighting chance of ending up about as bad as they were before surgery. On the other hand, most high-volume cataract surgeons will tell you that they simply do not see the type of problems that retina people fuss about. Who is right? Everyone, probably.

The older literature definitely suggests that cataract surgery is far less successful in diabetics than in non-diabetics. These reports were based on rather rambunctious surgical procedures, such as intracapsular or large-incision extracapsular surgery. Doctors who have lived through this era tend to be the most conservative about suggesting cataract surgery in diabetics.

Fortunately, the results tend to be much better with modern cataract surgery. In fact, some recent papers suggest that cataract surgery may have little or no effect on retinopathy progression for patients with minimal disease. The aggressive use of laser treatment to stabilize the retina has also helped improve results. Perhaps the most important factor is the much better systemic control that patients have nowadays.

However, because studies suggesting the safety of modern surgery are not large, controlled studies with long-term follow up, there is no way to rule out a subtle effect on retinopathy acceleration after cataract surgery. So proceed with an open mind—you may feel that *your* surgery would never make a diabetic worse, but we just don't know that such an assertion will remain true over many years. Besides, no matter how reassuring the modern literature may be, there is no doubt that some diabetic eyes will crash—even after perfect surgery.

Although there are no large trials that tell us exactly who will get into trouble, there are some basic rules to follow. First of all, recognize that even if you are awesome at doing phacos, you will have a few patients who end up with progression of their diabetic retinopathy. You therefore must warn all diabetics about the possible consequences, even if you think retina specialists are a bunch of overprotective weenies.

It helps to think of a diabetic's eye in terms of plumbing. A new house with shiny new pipes can handle a lot of abuse. An old house with pipes that are about to rust through will do OK if you take it really easy, but if you hammer away on them or crank up the pressure, you will blow everything out. The blood vessels in diabetic eyes with even a little bit of retinopathy can behave like rusty pipes. They seem to be very sensitive to increases in inflammatory mediators, and

By the way, none of this applies if you are trying to do cataract surgery in a developing country, where patients are likely to have poor control and fragile retinopathy. Under these circumstances, surgery is much more likely to cause trouble and it makes sense to be as conservative as possible. This is especially true if your only option is to do a less gentle technique such as extracapsular surgery. You should also be ready to get in a bunch of laser as soon as you can visualize the retina so, hopefully, the eye doesn't get a chance to deteriorate.

every effort should be made to perform surgery as smoothly and gently as possible to avoid stressing the system. Do not try out new things on your diabetic patients—they need the benefit of your best surgical technique, not the latest micro-incision phaco that your surgical rep is dying to show you. Anything that results in more intraocular manipulation and damage will greatly increase the risk of postoperative retinopathy progression. Repeat: If there are any problems during the surgery—even something mild like scruffing up the iris with your phaco tip—you have to watch extra carefully for retinopathy progression postoperatively.

Assuming you can provide smooth, state-of-the-art surgery for your patient, you still cannot be sure that all diabetics will do well. Your goal should be to identify those patients whose eyes may be microvascular booby-traps so that neither you nor the patient is unpleasantly surprised. Here are some things to consider:

Patients who seem to do best are usually either at the very beginning or at the very end of their retinopathy careers. In other words, patients with only minimal disease (maybe less than a few scattered microaneurysms and blot hemorrhages) tend to do well. Patients with quiescent, treated retinopathy also tend to do well. These are the patients who have taken good care of their diabetes and have a history of laser treatment that has stabilized their retinopathy for many years. This does not guarantee that such patients will do well—bad things can still happen to these burned-out eyes when you least expect it. As a general rule, though, patients with stable treated disease have much better odds than patients with active disease.

Because patients with minimal disease tend to do better, there are occasional cataract-ists who suggest that one should be even more aggressive about doing surgery in such patients. The thinking is that one should get the incipient cataract out of there now—when the eye can tolerate it better and the odds of safe surgery are better. It is argued that if one waits years for the cataract to get worse, then the retinopathy will also be getting worse, and the chance for successful surgery is diminished. This thinking is not unreasonable.

Guess what? There is no definite data that either supports or refutes this supposition. The problem is that the only way to find out whether "pre-emptive" cataract surgery is a good idea would be to randomize diabetics with early cataracts to either have surgery or not have surgery, and then follow them for years to see if the operated group has more rapid progression. Such a study is not likely to occur any time soon.

It is definitely not a good idea to operate on anyone's cataracts just because "they will be getting worse anyway." That is a potentially slippery slope. On the other hand, you may feel justified in operating on diabetic patients with mild cataract symptoms and minimal retinopathy in order to avoid waiting for both problems to get worse. Your judgment of the patient's situation and your personal results with such patients are your best guide. Do be sure to look for all the warning signs outlined in this chapter, though, and be prepared for the occasional unpleasant surprise…

Be very careful of patients whose retinopathy is in the "middle"—those who do not have very early disease or old burned-out disease. Someone with lots of microaneurysms and exudates in the posterior pole—even if there is no significant thickening—can really take off after cataract surgery. The same is true for patients with severe nonproliferative retinopathy, and it is especially true if such patients appear to be on the brink of needing treatment or if their retinopathy is not completely controlled by laser they have already had. If there is any doubt that the patient's retinopathy may be problematic, you may want to have the patient evaluated preoperatively by a retina specialist to cover yourself.

It goes without saying (so why is it being said?) that any pre-existing macular edema or proliferative disease should be aggressively treated prior to cataract surgery. In fact, you should have a low threshold for treating disease that you might not otherwise treat. For instance, a patient with some macular edema that is not clinically significant may benefit from treatment prior to cataract surgery. Or, you may consider doing preoperative PRP on a patient with severe NPDR whom you might otherwise just observe. It would be nice if you could wait a few months after any laser before doing cataract surgery in order to let the eye settle down and to be sure that everything is really stable.

If the cataract is bad enough that you can't easily perform accurate focal treatment, it is at least reasonable to try to get some grid treatment in. This does require special care because in order to squeak through the cataract you will be using smaller spots and higher powers, and the scattering of the beam may vary greatly from spot to spot. You need to watch your aiming beam closely, and if it suddenly snaps into focus, you have to turn the power down to avoid rupturing Bruch's membrane. (You can also use some of the techniques described in Chapter 9 to control the fluence without having to reach over and change the laser settings every five seconds.) This is where the ability to use an indirect contact lens can greatly facilitate treatment, allowing you to more easily work around the media opacities. Panretinal photocoagulation through a cataract tends to be less tricky; it is more "meatball" in nature, and you can usually work around the opacities and get at least a partial treatment in.

Interestingly, there is a recent paper suggesting that patients with severe nonproliferative disease or non-high-risk proliferative disease may have less trouble with postoperative macular edema if their PRP is performed *after* cataract surgery, rather than before it.[1] The authors postulate that this may be a function of subclinical inflammation caused by the PRP, which is then exacerbated by subsequent cataract surgery. The study needs to be confirmed by large studies—there is still a strong sense that it is better to get any retinopathy under control with laser prior to surgery. This data does, however, support the concept of waiting at least a few months after a laser before doing cataract surgery in order to give things time to settle down.

The real point is that, once again, something that is considered an absolute truth may change with time. Keep your eyes and mind open…

In addition to pretreatment with laser, it is reasonable to use preoperative non-steroidals and aggressive postoperative nonsteroidals and topical steroids in these patients—and to continue such treatment a month or two longer than one would in a non-diabetic. Such treatment helps to blunt the deleterious effects of perioperative inflammation on the fragile diabetic vasculature.

Finally, when it comes to preoperative treatments, more and more specialists are considering intravitreal bevacizumab or triamcinolone to better control the retinopathy at the time of surgery. Because there are no definitive guidelines for using these drugs for retinopathy in general, there are certainly no guidelines for using them in this setting. However, they may be useful in eyes with metastable macular edema in order to protect the macula from progression. The approach here is so variable that if you are at all worried about your patient's retina, you really should quiz your local retinal community about how to proceed.

Another "well, duh" point is to keep in mind the visual potential of the eye. If the patient has had macular edema or macular traction, you cannot expect them to have excellent results, and you must really warn the patient about this. Even if they only have minimal retinopathy, remember that diabetes can affect retinal functioning in ways that aren't identified by Snellen acuity or glare testing. In other words, your experience with non-diabetic cataracts has taught you that your surgery will eliminate a host of symptoms. However, even fairly normal-looking diabetic retinas have subtle problems with, for instance, decreased contrast sensitivity or dark adaptation. These subtle defects mean that taking the cataract out will not be as likely to eliminate their symptoms as it would be in non-diabetics. Both you and the patient need to alter your expectations in recognition of this.

You may not fully appreciate how important it is for both the surgeon and the patient to have appropriate expectations until you have your first diabetic patient burst into tears when they realize that they still have retinal problems, even though they just had cataract surgery. Patients have a strong tendency to assume that everything will be great as soon as that cataract is popped out, and they are especially likely to think this if their vision is already a bit blurry from retinopathy. The success of cataract surgery in the general population has created such a high level of expectation that patients imagine the cataract is causing all of their problems—in spite of having had everything covered in this book explained to them again and again.

You have to specifically discuss with patients the fact that they may be disappointed, even if the surgery goes perfectly—even if they have only minimal retinopathy and even if the retinopathy does not progress. The patient's thinking may be wildly unrealistic in spite of careful counseling—for instance, they may think that cataract surgery will somehow eliminate all of their retinopathy, as well. These kinds of thoughts will likely go unvoiced, so you need to anticipate them and ask about their expectations in order to make sure the two of you are thinking the same thing.

By the same token, you should not let yourself become delusional about the visual potential of an eye or the visual significance of a cataract. It is easy to look at a mild diabetic cataract and apply the same criteria you would for a non-diabetic, ignoring the retinal pitfalls that may exist. Be sure you are familiar with the patient's vision prior to the development of the cataract; then you will not be fooled when a mildly damaged retina—and not a mild lens opacity—is the real culprit. And definitely don't be fooled by the kind of dramatic cortical cataracts that diabetics sometimes have—these can look terrible, but they tend to be visually insignificant.

Should you perform a routine preoperative fluorescein angiogram or OCT on diabetic patients who are being considered for cataract surgery? Most retina specialists would answer in the affirmative, because you get a lot of information that helps to predict the likelihood for trouble in the postoperative period. The OCT can reveal subtle thickening, warning you that the retina is just barely handling the leakage present. It will also demonstrate subtle epiretinal membranes that may contract postoperatively and create the need for a vitrectomy. The angiogram will give you an idea about pre-existing capillary dropout near the fovea, something that suggests the eye is quite fragile—even if the vision is still good. If there is a lot of macular ischemia on the angiogram, then it is likely that any cataract present is not visually significant at all. An angiogram can also demonstrate subtle diffuse leakage that, even if it has not yet caused retinal thickening, may lead to macular edema after the leakage is revved up by post-op inflammatory mediators.

This is not to say that preoperative fluorescein angiography and OCT are mandatory. You may be in a situation where such testing is not readily available, or you may feel that the clinical exam is so good that no testing is needed. The point is that if you have even a remote concern that occult retinopathy may be lying in wait, you should consider these tests. This is especially true about performing an OCT—there is no morbidity involved in doing an OCT, and you should have a very low threshold for doing this test if you have one.

Another crucial preoperative factor is the degree of the patient's control. You *cannot* ignore this. Your training has taught you to meticulously evaluate refractive issues, IOL selection, and biometry with all the conscientiousness you can muster. But if you do not ask about the patient's hemoglobin A1c and blood pressure, you are being as irresponsible as if you were to select the IOL power by drawing numbers out of a hat. Here's why:

There are some studies that suggest poor control is not highly correlated with postoperative progression, at least in the short term, but there are other studies indicating that bad control will clearly contribute to loss of vision and progressive retinopathy after surgery. (Murtha and Cavallarano provide a nice review of all this.[2]) Ultimately, you have to recognize that ignoring a patient's poor control will result in a worse outcome—even if the cataract surgery had nothing to do with it.

Look at it this way—A tremendous amount of effort is devoted to preventing endophthalmitis, and rightly so. Massive editorials and reviews are written trying to identify nuances that can shave a few tenths of a percentage point off the incidence. People agonize (and drug companies battle) over which prophylactic drops to use as well as other factors, such as the surgical prep and construction of the wound. Heck, if that cataract guru in Florida said that he had eliminated endophthalmitis over the last 20,000 cases by having patients eat broccoli the night before surgery, you know you would try it.

All this is well and good, but go back to Figure 2 in Chapter 20 and look at how much a hemoglobin A1c of 9% can mess up the results of even perfect surgery. Even if one postulates that the level of control does not affect the surgical results per se (and it is hard to believe that it doesn't), one has to admit that in the long run patients who have cataract surgery and have good control will do far better than patients who have cataract surgery and have poor control.

Endophthalmitis is bad, of course. However, one almost never stops to realize that over time the visual results of operating on a poorly controlled diabetic's cataract are likely to be poor. Most endophthalmitis, if caught early and treated aggressively, will have a better outcome than the vision that results from a fovea ruined by macular edema. In other words, do go ahead and fight endophthalmitis, but recognize that exercising restraint with diabetic cataracts and having patients take the time to get tuned-up systemically will give your diabetic patients far better results compared to the microscopic change in risk that may or may not exist when you jump on the latest pre-op antibiotic train. Even orthopedic surgeons have to take some responsibility for the rest of the patient. You can, too.

There is yet another reason to make the patient's overall control as much a part of your pre-op eval as the slit lamp exam and keratometry. As mentioned in Chapter 20, patients may have temporary worsening of their retinopathy when they try to improve their control. It turns out that if a patient with poor control decides to improve their control at the same time that they have cataract surgery, they can end up with marked postoperative worsening of their retinopathy.[3]
Does this mean that you should encourage any patient with bad control to continue being bad for a few months after cataract surgery? Only if you are a buccaneer trying to jack up your surgery volume at all costs. It seems far better to wait several months for the patient to get better control and then do the surgery. The point, again, is that if you are not aware of the patient's control when you recommend surgery, you have blown off a variable that may be more important than any other part of the ophthalmic exam. Remember, if you screw up an IOL, you can fix them with glasses, Lasik or an IOL exchange. If you screw up someone's macula, it is gone forever.

What about patients with bilateral cataracts?

It is probably not a good idea to operate on both eyes of a patient with bilateral cataracts and worrisome retinopathy within a brief period of time, if you can possibly help it. If the patient is going to get into trouble, it may take two to three months for it to show up, and you may want to wait this long before doing the second eye. There are many patients who prefer their 20/50 cataract to their nice shiny implant because their macula folded up after surgery.

What is the best IOL?

The best IOL is usually the one that you can put in best. (Bestly?) Again, your diabetic patient is not the one on whom to try some slinky new IOL from the rep; just use the tools that allow you to do your safest surgery. Some papers recommend using a lens with a large optic; this will allow better visualization in case the patient ends up needing extensive laser or a vitrectomy. It is also helpful if the patient has a larger capsulotomy, especially given the tendency for diabetic capsules to contract after surgery. These are good ideas if you can do them safely, but not if you have to totally change your technique.

There has also been discussion about whether such patients should get a silicone IOL. There is no question that a silicone IOL can be a real pain during vitrectomy surgery due to condensation that occurs whenever the eye is filled with air. Also, if the patient needs silicone oil to repair their retina, it pretty much guarantees that the IOL will need to be exchanged, because the oil will ruin it. However, the need to perform these maneuvers is relatively unlikely and it is hard to know which patient will get into trouble—unless the patient has horrible retinopathy that is not well controlled. As a result, if you do your best surgery with a silicone IOL, by all means, use a silicone IOL. On the other hand, if you think the patient may be heading into trouble, it might be helpful to use a more "retina-friendly" acrylic IOL—this will be less problematic if the patient does end up needing a vitrectomy. Ultimately, you know far more about IOLs than most retina doctors and you should do what you think is safest. If, however, you are using a silicone IOL simply because it is the cheapest option for your surgery center—well, perhaps you need to clean out the part of your brain that manufactures rationalizations…

Multifocal IOLs are a bit more problematic. You need a perfectly functioning macula to handle a multifocal IOL, and even if your diabetic patient has no obvious retinopathy, there may be subclinical defects in retinal function that can make adjusting to such an IOL much more difficult than you might expect. (Vide supra about how diabetics can have problems with contrast sensitivity that can affect their happiness with even a monofocal IOL.) Plus, if they get any retinopathy progression at all they will have even more problems. Flexible accommodating IOLs (such as the Crystalens) may have an advantage because they do not depend on crisp macular function, but they may not provide as much near vision, and a diabetic capsule can be quirky. The bottom line is that there really is no data right now indicating how to use any of these lenses in patients with diabetes. If you decide to use a presbyopia correcting lens, you need to proceed with caution, and both you and the patient need to be aware of the possible pitfalls.

What about doing a YAG?

There is no clear consensus on whether performing YAG laser capsulotomy can stir up retinopathy. It probably does not have much of an effect but, as usual, there are never any guarantees. If you have to do a lot of hacking and slashing with the YAG you may cause enough inflammation to affect the retina, especially if the patient has already had complicated cataract surgery. It probably makes sense to put diabetics on some sort of anti-inflammatory drop around the time of the laser—more laser or more preexisting damage may mean more topical therapy.

Perhaps the most important thing is to not talk yourself into doing a YAG on "trace" capsular opacities when the patient is dropping to 20/50 from subtle macular edema that you are missing. Never give up your fundamental job of looking for all the potential causes of vision loss.

What if, in spite of the best intentions, the macula blows out after your excellent cataract surgery?

If the macula swells up after surgery, one traditionally follows a stepwise approach. First of all, continue aggressive topical therapy with non-steroidal and steroid drops to treat any pseudophakic component to the edema. Laser any obvious disease, but don't keep firing away until the fovea is a doughnut hole in the middle of a laser wasteland. It is easy to succumb to the temptation to keep lasering post-op edema, because it can keep on coming, but if treating the obvious leaks does not solve the problem you need to think pharmacologically and try a periocular steroid injection. This is particularly true if there is a lot of diffuse leakage and late staining of the optic nerve on angiography—these findings suggest that postoperative inflammation is driving the vascular leakage rather than pure diabetic disease. In such cases, it may be best to go sooner to a periocular steroid injection to try to control the process.

If drops, laser, and a periocular shot don't fix things quickly, it is likely that your patient will be getting a bit frustrated. This is where intravitreal triamcinolone can save the day—assuming there are no complications from the injection. Some retina specialists advocate foregoing a stepwise approach altogether and, instead, simply initiating treatment with intravitreal steroids to get rapid control of the edema (and to get rapid control of the patient's patience). Intravitreal steroids clearly have more risk—see Chapter 11—and whether you go with the stepped approach or you go straight to intravitreal therapy depends on how bad the edema is and how much risk you and the patient are willing to accept to get better, faster. (Intravitreal bevacizumab may be another option—there is less chance of a pressure rise, but recall that the drug seems to be less effective in general.)

As always, watch out for subtle epiretinal membranes or vitreomacular traction—an OCT is crucial in this setting. If traction-related pathology is present it is very unlikely that intravitreal treatment—or anything short of a vitrectomy—will have a significant effect. Such patients usually need referral to a retina specialist. Hopefully you explained the potential for this prior to surgery, and the patient is not vindictively disappointed by all the extra fuss.

Don't forget that other things can happen after surgery, such as a big vitreous hemorrhage or progressive traction as the vitreous shifts forward when the crystalline lens is removed. These problems usually need referral to determine whether the patient needs surgery to protect their vision. One hopes that this will never happen to you because you will have treated everything and made sure the retina is stable before surgery—but never underestimate the ability of diabetes to scramble up your best-laid plans.

By now, you should be getting the impression that a patient with diabetes and a cataract needs to be on a totally separate track relative to a patient with just a cataract. Here are a few other things to think about:

In addition to being more aggressive with perioperative topical therapy, you should also be more aggressive with your follow up. If the macula swells it tends to do so after several weeks, and if you see the patient a couple of times in the first month and then send them off for glasses you can miss it. Also, the macula is more likely to start swelling as the drops are tapered. If you give the patient some sort of automatic tapering schedule and don't check them yourself you can miss early changes that could be easily treated—and then they will come in when they have definite symptoms with advanced disease that will be harder to control.

This is especially true if you are doing the co-management thing. You must make sure that the optometrist who will follow the patient knows how to watch for early changes in the fundus appearance that suggest trouble is brewing and that they will follow the patient closer than a typical post-op cataract patient if you can't.

Note: In order to avoid a lot of polemics, it is worth pointing out that the preceding paragraph is not meant to necessarily condone co-management. Rather, it simply recognizes that co-management is a reality, and can be a reasonable compromise in situations where distance, cost and time preclude personal follow up on what is usually a routine and uncomplicated surgical procedure. The point is that you need to remember that diabetics should not be left on the assembly-line portion of your cataract factory. They really need to be taken off the line and brought over to the custom shop for closer attention.

Finale

To review: Modern-day cataract surgery is much safer relative to older tech-niques, and generally does not seem to stir things up much in terms of retin-opathy progression. On the other hand, there are patients who can still do very poorly, but you have a fighting chance of weeding such patients out by using your noggin. Watch out for the level of retinopathy and for the stability of the retinopathy. Have a low threshold for doing a pre-op OCT and fluorescein an-giogram, and consider sending the patient out for a retina consult if necessary. Know the patient's degree of systemic control. Know the likely visual potential of the eye, and make darn sure the patient understands the limits and extra risks inherent with cataract surgery in diabetics. Do the best surgery you can, and then watch the patient closely afterwards. Don't hesitate to ask for help if prob-lems arise. Unfortunately, the secretary will *not* disavow any knowledge of your actions, so be careful.

Finale to the Finale

There is one other issue that doesn't quite fit in anywhere else—and that is what happens in a patient's mind when one simply mentions that they have a "cataract." Diabetic patients may fixate on this information to a surprising de-gree, and this can be particularly true if the cataract is not visually significant and you have no intention of doing anything about it. The problem is that even if you tell them their cataract is insignificant, they will often assign any visual symptoms they have to the cataract whether or not this is the actual case. This means they will ignore new symptoms on the assumption that they stem from "a simple cataract," and will then assume that they can address the problem whenever they have time.

Unfortunately, if their symptoms are from retinal disease, they may end up with irreversible vision loss while they wait to find a convenient time to fit an eye exam into their schedule. As a result of this, many retina docs have a vague reluctance to even talk about cataracts at all unless they are definitely visually significant.* This scenario is not limited to diabetic retinopathy; it can happen with any retinal disease, and it is especially common with macular degeneration.

The real message here is that if you discuss the presence of a cataract, you need to clearly spell out to the patient that they should not diagnose them-selves if their vision gets worse. If they notice a definite change it is unlikely to be from the cataract, and they need to get back in quickly to avoid perma-nent vision loss.

*Of course, retina specialists do have to mention cataracts—even if they aren't relevant. If a patient with a visually insignificant cataract ends up go-ing to a more anteriorly oriented doctor—who *will* mention the cataract—the patient will think the retina specialist is useless for not being the first to talk about it.

References and Suggested Reading

1.   Suto C, Hori S, Kato S. Management of type 2 diabetics requiring panretinal photocoagulation and cataract surgery. J Cataract Refract Surg 2008;34:1001-6.

2.   Murtha T, Cavallerano J. The management of diabetic eye disease in the setting of cataract surgery. Curr Opin Ophthalmol 2007;18:13-8.

3.   Suto C, Hori S, Kato S, Muraoka K, Kitano S. Effect of perioperative glycemic control in progression of diabetic retinopathy and maculopathy. Arch Ophthalmol 2006;124:38-45.

Tsujikawa A, Otani A, Takanashi T, Ogura Y. Long-term prognosis of extracapsular cataract extraction and intraocular lens implantation in diabetic patients. Jpn J Ophthalmol 1997;41:319-23.

Jaffe GJ, Burton TC, Kuhn E, Prescott A, Hartz A. Progression of nonproliferative diabetic retinopathy and visual outcome after extracapsular cataract extraction and intraocular lens implantation. Am J Ophthalmol 1992;114:448-56.

Romero-Aroca P, Fernandez-Ballart J, Almena-Garcia M, Mendez-Marin I, Salvat-Serra M, Buil-Calvo JA. Nonproliferative diabetic retinopathy and macular edema progression after phacoemulsification: prospective study. J Cataract Refract Surg 2006;32:1438-44.

Chew EY, Benson WE, Remaley NA, et al. Results after lens extraction in patients with diabetic retinopathy: early treatment diabetic retinopathy study report number 25. Arch Ophthalmol 1999;117:1600-6.

Squirrell D, Bhola R, Bush J, Winder S, Talbot JF. A prospective, case controlled study of the natural history of diabetic retinopathy and maculopathy after uncomplicated phacoemulsification cataract surgery in patients with type 2 diabetes. Br J Ophthalmol 2002;86:565-71.

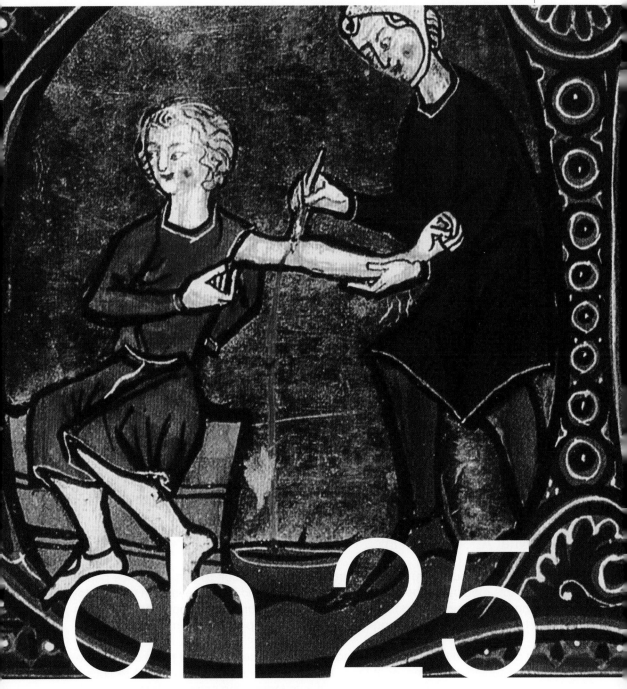

ch 25

A Thinning of the Blood

Co-Author: James E. Schmidt, M.D., F.A.C.C

One issue that often arises is whether it is safe to use aspirin in the setting of proliferative diabetic retinopathy—both the patient and their internist have visions of torrents of intraocular blood. Fortunately, the Early Treatment Diabetic Retinopathy Study clearly showed that aspirin does not make any difference in any aspect of diabetic retinopathy, and in particular, does not increase the risk for vitreous hemorrhages.[1] You can reassure patients that if they need to be on aspirin for other medical problems, it really does not affect their ophthalmic disease. By the way, you are not alone if you think this result seems horribly counterintuitive. It is hard to imagine that the same patients who show you all the bruises on their forearms from taking aspirin have absolutely no increased amount of hemorrhage from the ratty vessels in their eyes. Perhaps the vitreous changes the need for functioning platelets, or perhaps the nature of the abnormal vessels is such that alterations in platelet activity aren't important. No one knows. Whatever the reason, you have one big whopping study behind you to reassure both the patient and the patient's internist that they can use aspirin with impunity.

What about other antiplatelet agents such as ticlopidine (Ticlid) and clopidogrel (Plavix)?

There are no massive studies looking at the effect of these drugs on diabetic retinopathy as there is for aspirin. However, as far as anyone can tell they don't seem to have a significant impact on diabetic retinopathy, so they are probably as benign as aspirin. "Probably" is the key word, though. Because their use isn't supported by the kind of data that supports the use of aspirin, no one can say that they are absolutely equivalent in terms of risk. In other words, you can tell patients on these other drugs that because aspirin is OK, and because these drugs are similar, it is likely that there are no ill effects—but there are no guarantees. (Check the blue box on the facing page for one other concern.)

What About Warfarin?

Warfarin (Coumadin) can sometimes be more difficult to sort out. Once patients on this medication hear that they could get blood in their eye from retinopathy, they (and their doctors) will become rightfully concerned about the use of this drug. This issue takes more finesse than the aspirin question.

If patients are placed on Coumadin, it is because they need to be on it for life-threatening problems, or at least, that is what one would assume. A tedious but conscientious step is to make sure this is indeed the case by checking with the prescribing physician. Certain medical problems mandate the use of Coumadin (i.e., atrial fibrillation or recent deep venous thrombosis). Other times, patients may have been placed on Coumadin for more vague indications, and you may even find occasional patients who were left on the drug because no one took the time to decide whether they still needed it. This may be especially true if you practice in an area that is away from high-powered academic or "big city" medical groups. Please forgive the following generalization, but if the patient is being closely followed by a medical subspecialist for a recent problem, the odds are that everything is being done properly.

> **Important safety tip:**
>
> If you grew up in the old days, you may have become used to the idea that patients are on aspirin and/or Plavix for "general maintenance," and that such drugs can easily be stopped on a temporary basis. It turns out that it is usually not necessary to stop such drugs for typical ophthalmic surgeries—but sometimes doctors will do it because the perceived risk of discontinuing the drug is thought to be small and they feel safer doing surgery without it on board. It may be possible to do this for brief periods under certain circumstances—but you should check with the patient's doctor if you feel you must stop it.
>
> This is because nowadays there is a very good reason to *not* stop these medications at all. Patients may be on Plavix (or Ticlid) and aspirin because a drug-eluting stent has been placed in one or more of their coronary arteries. Discontinuing these drugs in this situation carries a definite risk of thrombosis, even if the drugs are stopped for only a short period of time. (These stents are slow to endothelialize.) Usually patients have been warned about this and they will make a big fuss if you casually suggest stopping the drugs, but one can never depend on this. You need to specifically ask about why they are on the drugs, and you should never stop such medications without getting clearance (and in this case, you may not be allowed to stop the drugs).
>
> The problem is that often decisions about these medications are made by checking off boxes on the patient's surgical scheduling form at a time when it is difficult to track down all the necessary information. If you really feel you need to change these medications, you must take the time to review the situation with the patient's medical specialists before making any recommendations.

If, however, the patient has been given Coumadin for some time by a non-specialist, and for what sounds like a dodgy indication (i.e., "My doctor says my arteries are hardening and I need thinner blood"), you may want to make a quick call to learn the real scoop. Your patient may be quite grateful (and will definitely have less morbidity) if you uncover a situation in which Coumadin can be decreased or discontinued safely—and no one would have realized it unless you took the effort.

If, however, the patient is being treated appropriately, there is another thing you should consider even though it is something you may have sworn you would never do again once you finished your internship. If a patient presents with an acute vitreous hemorrhage (or any ocular hemorrhage, for that matter), you should have a very low threshold for actually filling out a lab slip and checking the patient's INR. With the advent of anticoagulation clinics most patients are well maintained, but sometimes a patient's INR can go up unexpectedly. If patients are being treated outside of such clinics, there is a chance that their INR may not have been monitored for some time. Either way, if their blood happens to be really thin, you might save them from a massive hemorrhage somewhere else.

You will also be called on to decide how risky it is for a patient to begin or to continue Coumadin. Many internal medicine specialists have been taught that proliferative diabetic retinopathy and/or a vitreous hemorrhage are close to absolute contraindications to Coumadin. Your patient with a vitreous hemorrhage may suddenly be taken off the drug when they need it to keep from, well, dying. More commonly, the patient may decide to stop the drug on their own. If the patient has had relatively quiescent retinopathy, you might save their life by taking the time to explain to both the treating physician and the patient that retinopathy is at most a relative contraindication to anticoagulation.

Even if their retinal disease is problematic, it usually takes second fiddle to their systemic need for Coumadin, and the nuances of this may require a direct conversation with the anticoagulationist: You know the eye situation and the other doctor knows the patient's systemic disease, and some sort of mind meld can usually be achieved. Moreover, the intermittent and unexpected nature of diabetic hemorrhages needs to be conveyed to the internist. They are often thinking in terms of short-term hemorrhagic problems (like a GI bleed), and they need to know that the course of diabetic retinopathy is usually unpredictable and sporadic, and not something that tends to go away after briefly stopping anticoagulation just one time.

Oh yeah, and don't forget to include the patient in all this. First of all, most patients assume that the Coumadin actually causes hemorrhages in their eye. You can use this as an opportunity to once again explain that hemorrhages are part of proliferative diabetic retinopathy and that Coumadin does not cause hemorrhages (although if a hemorrhage does occur, it may be more pronounced if the patient is on the medication). Then, you need to review with them the real issue: whether they are willing to risk their well-being by having a stroke or a pulmonary embolism, versus the theoretical risk of having more of a hemorrhage in their eye. Most of the time they understand and opt to be on Coumadin.

Some patients will not want to have anything to do with the drug, however, and this is certainly well within their rights; you just have to make sure they are making the decision based on the correct information. The point is that although the overall risk-to-benefit ratio strongly favors the use of Coumadin in patients with proliferative disease, you cannot ignore the fact that the patient needs to be involved in the decision and you need to document the discussion in the same way one would document a surgical consent. Because…

...**from the standpoint of a retinal surgeon,** patients on Coumadin can, on occasion, be problematic. Most of the time the tendency to hemorrhage to a greater degree, if present, can be handled with laser and/or vitrectomy and there is no problem at all with the anticoagulation. Sometimes, though, they just keep bleeding, and they need an eye full of silicone oil to be able to see. This is not common, but it is a potential outcome that, for instance, may approach the risk of a stroke in the mind of a patient who is on Coumadin because of atrial fibrillation. As a comprehensive ophthalmologist, this is not likely to be a problem you will have to face. Still, it is important to realize that some patients may feel that the risk of Coumadin to the eyes begins to equal the systemic morbidity that the Coumadin is being used to prevent.

Incidentally, as mentioned in Chapter 12, a patient's need to be on Coumadin is another factor that may lead you to be more aggressive about treating severe nonproliferative diabetic retinopathy. It can be argued that early treatment may prevent any proliferative disease and thereby really minimize the risk of recurrent hemorrhage. (Remember, even involuted neovascularization may bleed from traction—and if there was never any neo in the first place you can sidestep the whole problem.) There is no data in the literature that specifically looks at this, but it is certainly something to consider in your decision to treat. The whole reason patients come to you instead of the PRP machine at Wal-Mart is because you can individualize the treatment rather than blindly follow a rulebook. No pun intended.

What about thrombolytics?

You have no doubt been contacted by the interventional cardiologist on call about a patient who needs acute thrombolysis or heparin. Once again, the life-threatening nature of the problem trumps the eye, but the patient still deserves some sort of informed consent. It turns out that the literature suggests that most of the time patients with proliferative retinopathy will do well. For instance, the GUSTO-I trial (Global Utilization of Streptokinase and t-PA for Occluded coronary arteries – I) had no intraocular hemorrhages among 6,011 patients with diabetes, and about 300 of those patients had proliferative retinopathy.[2] Still, there is possibility that patients could have a hemorrhage, and they deserve to be informed of the theoretical risk—but it is hard to imagine why they would not have thrombolytics if they are indicated.

What about operating on patients who are on Coumadin?

It is well accepted that it is OK to do modern cataract surgery on uncomplicated, anticoagulated patients.[3] Retinal surgery—or even complicated anterior segment surgery—is more likely to have problems with bleeding and there is no definitive study that provides a solid answer. Furthermore, you can be screwed no matter what you do: If you stop the Coumadin and the patient has a pulmonary embolism or a stroke, there will always be some hired-gun "expert" to say you should have done something differently. If you don't stop the Coumadin and the patient has a choroidal hemorrhage that destroys the eye, there will always be some hired-gun "expert" to say you should have done something differently. You can't win unless you put in some thoughtful pre-op face time.

There is a growing feeling in the retina community that it is OK to continue Coumadin (and anti-platelet agents) when patients need retinal surgery. The ocular risk in general is thought to be less than the systemic risk posed by stopping the drug.[4, 5] (You still need to know the INR at the time of surgery, though—if it is way high, you are taking risks you shouldn't take.)

Another option is to switch to shorter-acting heparin derivatives, such as enoxaparin (Lovenox), and stopping everything just before surgery and restarting it afterward. This involves a lot of expense and hassle. However, if you are treating a patient with a lot of hemorrhagic potential, this may be something to consider because, again, the potential risk of an intraoperative hemorrhage in the mind of such a patient (e.g., a one-eyed smoker who has high myopia and severe proliferative disease that may also need a scleral buckle) may be equal to the systemic risk of being off anticoagulation.

A final option, and perhaps the most commonly used one if it is felt that Coumadin is a problem, is to stop the drug a few days before surgery so that there is still a slight antocoagulative effect but hopefully not enough to affect the case. This last approach is somewhat vague and unscientific, but it generally seems to be an accepted compromise.

Ultimately, if you think anticoagulation may represent a risk to the patient's surgery, you simply have to bite the bullet and use your most valuable commodity—time—and communicate with the patient and the anticoagulationist treating the patient. This is true whether you want to stop the drug or not. The patient must understand that although we think it is acceptable to do complex surgery with Coumadin on board, there are no guarantees, and they must also understand the risk of stopping the Coumadin and having a stroke (or whatever disease the Coumadin is preventing). The anticoagulationist must know what your ophthalmic concerns are—sometimes they are surprisingly content with stopping the Coumadin, and sometimes they are adamant about continuing it (or doing the Lovenox thing, for instance, if the patient has a mechanical valve).

Remember that you are the only doctor in the mix who understands what can happen to an eye, and you *will* be responsible. So don't play the sleazy ophthalmology game of "Well, the cardiologist said it was OK to stop it because he signed a form letter, so I don't have to think about this." You have to decide what can go wrong with the eye and how much risk you are willing to balance by continuing or not continuing the Coumadin—and then you really have to work with everyone to come up with a plan. If something goes wrong, at least everyone will feel that they were warned and they were given a chance to think about the ramifications of their choices.

Basically, we are spoiled because we routinely get away with both starting and stopping Coumadin and/or operating on anticoagulated patients without having any problems. It is therefore easy to become complacent about the drug and to forget that if something does go wrong, there will be plenty of people ready to second-guess all of your actions. You should review the possible concerns with any patient on Coumadin because you want the patient to have heard about the issues well before, heaven forbid, something bad happens.

Of all the chapters in this book, this one is perhaps the diciest, because it involves decisions regarding systemic factors that are well beyond the expertise of even the most renaissance ophthalmologist. Please recognize that the medical doctors caring for these patients have devoted their lives to understanding the risks and benefits of anticoagulation and you should be ready to discuss problematic patients on an individual basis with them. Under no circumstances should you consider the brief overview here to represent a definitive guide about how to manage such patients.

If you need further information there are very useful reviews found at UpTo-Date.com—an exhaustive internet database that covers all aspects of this subject as well as most of medicine. A lot of the information here is abstracted from that source.

Also, recognize that there is a significant literature concerning the risks of anticoagulation relative to surgery within each subspecialty of ophthalmology itself. An approach that works for routine cataract surgery may not work for high-risk glaucoma surgery. You should, of necessity, stay abreast of this information as it pertains to your own surgical practice.

What about doing a retrobulbar with Coumadin on board?

First, check the stuff in Chapter 15 about how to minimize pain using various laser settings, etc. If none of that works, then—surprise—there are no proven guidelines to follow. Here are some things to consider:

You can try a sub-Tenon's or subconjunctival block, also mentioned in Chapter 15. You can get pretty good anesthesia in the region you inject, and there is less chance for a globe-threatening hemorrhage. If you need to do 360 degrees of treatment, though, you can end up with a lot of tedious injections and these routes does not get as far back as you may need.

You can try more of a peribulbar approach, but it is not clear that this really protects you—if you are sticking needles in and around the orbit, you simply have to accept the risk of a big hemorrhage.

Basically, if you need to do some sort of orbital block, you have to once again use up your most valuable asset: time. You need to review with the patient the risks of a hemorrhage and the risk of delaying treatment in order to allow the Coumadin to wear off. You also need to review the risk of going off the Coumadin in terms of stroke or whatever the patient is on the stuff for. As alluded to above, it is usually not worth the risk to stop the drug for a simple retrobulbar.

Still, you should cover yourself by making sure that the INR is not way out of whack—it is a good idea to send the patient to the lab to check it or ask whether it has been checked in the recent past. Is there a value that is known to be safe for doing a retrobulbar? Of course not. No one has any "for sure" data. There is data from other specialties, however, that can be used to extrapolate the risk. You are "probably" safe if it is 2.0 or less. Indeed, you may want to let the anti-coagulationist know because this may mean the patient is sub-therapeutic.

If the patient is in the therapeutic range (usually 2.0 to 3.0), the literature suggests that it is OK to do, for instance, dental extractions, dermatologic procedures and routine cataract surgery, so this level may be acceptable for a retrobulbar, assuming the ocular indication warrants it.[6] The point is that you do not want to be doing a lateral cantholysis to decompress an orbital hemorrhage and then find out that the INR was 4.9 but you never checked it. As long as you make a conscientious effort to inform the patient of the risks and make sure the INR is not sky-high, you are doing a good job. Still—you should never become complacent about blocking patients on Coumadin, and you should recognize that the scales of risks and benefits can shift depending on why you need to do the block and the exact level of the INR.

> **Don't forget** to re-engage some of your atrophic clinical skills in this setting: Talk to and look at the patient. Someone with an INR of 2.1 and no problems with bruising or bleeding is very different from someone with an INR of 2.1 who is covered with bruises and sanguineous Band-Aids.

What about intravitreal injections?

There is more of a consensus that one does not need to worry about stopping anticoagulation at all in this setting—these are tiny needles going through a relatively avascular space, and raising the intraocular pressure with the injection is likely to mitigate any bleeding.[4] Should you check an INR? Most doctors don't—a history of stable anticoagulation seems to be enough. One can't argue against checking it—if you get into trouble you will wish you had checked it, but the logistics of sending every intravitreal injection patient down for a lab test and following up the results would be onerous, if not impossible. The odds are good that you will get away with doing nothing—but once again, don't forget to make sure the patient understands the risk they are taking so no one is surprised if Murphy and his Law appear.

> **While we are on the subject of thinned blood,** there is one other thing to consider. Don't forget to ask about herbal supplements in patients with ocular hemorrhages. For instance, ginkgo biloba in particular has been associated with spontaneous hyphema and retinal hemorrhages.[7] Garlic, ginseng and fish oil may also have anticoagulant properties or interact with anticoagulant medications.[8] It makes sense to be aware of any alternative therapies that patients may be taking.

References and suggested reading

1.   Effects of aspirin treatment on diabetic retinopathy. ETDRS report number 8. Early Treatment Diabetic Retinopathy Study Research Group. Ophthalmology 1991;98:757-65.

2.   Mahaffey KW, Granger CB, Toth CA, et al. Diabetic retinopathy should not be a contraindication to thrombolytic therapy for acute myocardial infarction: review of ocular hemorrhage incidence and location in the GUSTO-I trial. Global Utilization of Streptokinase and t-PA for Occluded Coronary Arteries. J Am Coll Cardiol 1997;30:1606-10.

3.   Barequet IS, Sachs D, Priel A, et al. Phacoemulsification of cataract in patients receiving Coumadin therapy: ocular and hematologic risk assessment. Am J Ophthalmol 2007;144:719-723.

4.   Charles S, Rosenfeld PJ, Gayer S. Medical consequences of stopping anticoagulant therapy before intraocular surgery or intravitreal injections. Retina 2007;27:813-5.

5.   Fu AD, McDonald HR, Williams DF, et al. Anticoagulation with warfarin in vitreoretinal surgery. Retina 2007;27:290-5.

6.   Douketis JD, Berger PB, Dunn AS, et al. The perioperative management of antithrombotic therapy: American College of Chest Physicians Evidence-Based Clinical Practice Guidelines (8th Edition). Chest 2008;133:299S-339S.

7.   Fraunfelder FW. Ocular side effects from herbal medicines and nutritional supplements. Am J Ophthalmol 2004;138:639-47.

8.   Spolarich AE, Andrews L. An examination of the bleeding complications associated with herbal supplements, antiplatelet and anticoagulant medications. J Dent Hyg 2007;81:67.

Carter JE. Anticoagulant, antiplatelet, and fibrinolytic (thrombolytic) therapy in patients at high risk for ocular hemorrhage. UpToDate.com, May 2008.

Lip GY. Management of anticoagulation before and after elective surgery. UpToDate.com, May 2008.

O'Donnell M, Kearon C. Perioperative management of oral anticoagulation. Cardiol Clin. 2008; 26:299-309.

Law SK, Song BJ, Yu F, Kurbanyan K, Yang TA, Caprioli J. Hemorrhagic complications from glaucoma surgery in patients on anticoagulation therapy or antiplatelet therapy. Am J Ophthalmol. 2008;145:736-746.

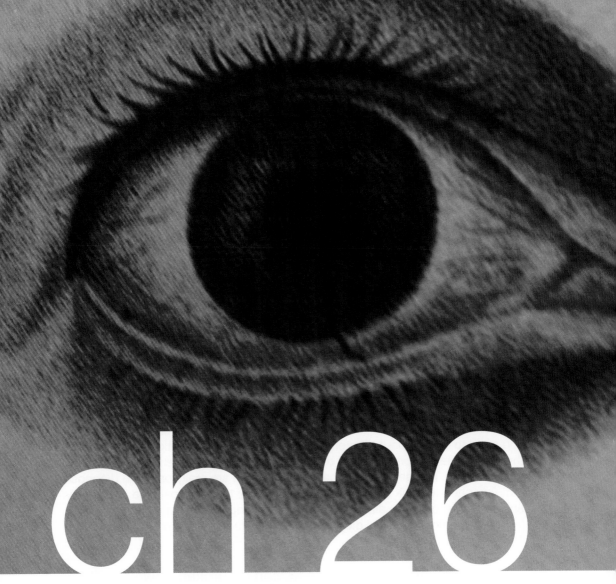

ch 26

Differential Diagnosis
A Rose Is a Rose Is Type 2a Juxtafoveal Telangiectasis

Usually you do not need to use your differential diagnosis powers with diabetic retinopathy, given that the patient already has the systemic diagnosis and the fundus findings are classic. This eliminates some brain strain but, as this book hopefully shows, the ease of diabetic diagnosis is more than made up for by the whole "art of medicine" thing. Still, you should never drop your guard completely, and you should always keep at least a little of your mental bandwidth available to think about the differential diagnosis because it sometimes make a big difference to you and your patient.

It is easy to come up with an inventory of things that can look like diabetic retinopathy—and the resulting lists are usually divided into, one, things that can make new blood vessels grow, and two, things that can make little hemorrhages and swollen capillaries show up all over the place.

Table 1 is an exhaustive look at the differential diagnosis of diseases that can make new blood vessels grow and can therefore simulate active proliferative retinopathy. It is one of the all-time classic tables from an equally classic paper by Jampol et al.[1]—a real keeper if you plan on doing a lot of retina, though you probably won't need it very much in the trenches of general ophthalmology. It is here for your edification.

Table 2 is typical of the standard list found in most texts for the differential diagnosis of background changes such as hemorrhages and microvascular abnormalities. You can scan it into your handheld and then you should be good to go for regurgitating facts on rounds, passing boards, impressing chicks and dudes at bars, etc., etc.

However, if you really want to be able to handle the Giant Smackdown of clinical life, you have to realize that reality tends to be more complex than mere tables. A list of diseases doesn't really give you a good matrix to work with, because you need to worry about different diseases in different situations. Remember that the whole reason to have a differential is to keep yourself and the patient out of trouble. A wise doctor once said that there are really only two diagnoses that you need to think of in any clinical situation: the diagnosis the patient has and the worst possible diagnosis if you are wrong. If want to explore the next level of diabetic differential diagnosis, feel free to read beyond the Land of the Tables…

The diabetic differential diagnosis can be broken down into three situations where you can screw up:

The first situation occurs when you have a patient with known retinopathy and a brand new disease shows up out of the blue. If the disease happens to be something that can look like diabetes, it can remain hidden within the preexisting retinopathy. Diseases such as these may be eminently treatable if you catch them in time, but they can make the patient much worse if you don't.

The second situation occurs in a patient with known diabetes but who, until

Table 1 / Differential Diagnosis of Peripheral Neovascularization

Vascular diseases with ischemia	
Sickling hemoglobinopathies	Other hemoglobinopathies
Eales' Disease	Branch retinal arteriolar occlusion
Small vessel hyalinosis	Retinal embolization
Diabetes mellitus	Retinopathy of prematurity
Branch retinal vein occlusion	Familial exudative vitreoretinopathy
Hyperviscosity syndromes	Toxemia of pregnancy
Aortic arch syndromes	Encircling buckling operation
Carotid-cavernous fistula	
Inflammatory diseases with possible ischemia	
Sarcoidosis	Retinal vasculitis
Uveities including pars planitis	Birdshot retinochoroidopathy
Toxoplasmosis	Acute retinal necrosis
Miscellaneous	
Incontentia pigmenti	Familial telanglectasia
Inheritied retinal venous beading	Cocaine abuse
Long-standing retinal detachment	Choroidal melanoma
Retinitis pigmentosa	Retinoschisis
Autosomal dominant vitreoretinochoroidopathy	

Table 2 / Differential Diagnosis of Background Diabetic Retinopathy

Radiation retinopathy	Juxtafoveal telangiectasis
Vein occlusions	Coats' disease
Ocular ischemic syndrome	Sickle cell retinopathy
Hypertensive retinopathy	Age-related microvascular changes
Hematologic abnormalities (anemia, leukemia, thrombocytopenia)	

now, has had no significant retinopathy. If said patient begins to get something funny in their retina, but it is not really diabetic disease, it is easy to call it diabetes and treat it incorrectly because you are blindfolded by the patient's systemic diagnosis.

The third situation is the typical one presented in most texts (and the purpose of tables such as those on the previous page). Namely, what should you think of if you have a patient who does not have known diabetes but has something that looks like diabetic retinopathy? This is fairly easy because you start by ruling out diabetes and then consider everything else covered in the above two situations.

> **Granted,** this categorization is artificial—these things can all overlap—so once you have internalized this knowledge don't go binary and forget that they can be combined in different ways (especially if your patient is unlucky). For instance, if you have a patient with retinopathy of unknown cause, and you skillfully diagnose diabetes, that patient can still get worse from a bunch of things that you are responsible for such as uveitis, a central retinal vein occlusion or, for that matter, sideroblastic anemia. Just don't ever stop thinking.

In any event, let's look at each one of these scenarios in greater detail.

Things that can hide in the signal-to-noise ratio of diabetic retinopathy and can make things worse if you don't think of them:

Diabetics are allowed to get other diseases, so if you are totally in the diabetic retinopathy zone you may fail to notice something crucial. Typically the new disease is missed because the superimposed findings are simply attributed to worsening of the underlying diabetic retinopathy. It is a Bad Thing to overlook such problems because if any other disease is added to diabetic retinopathy, the resulting synergy can be far worse than either entity alone.

One problem that can be hard to diagnose in the setting of retinopathy is uveitis. A rip-roaring HLA B-27 flare-up is easy to detect, but smoldering intermediate uveitis or retinal vasculitis can be hidden. For instance, if you think that every floating dot in your slit beam is just a red blood cell, you can miss white blood cells in the vitreous from intermediate uveitis. Or a subtle vasculitis can be mistaken for diabetes-related vascular changes (and there is no doubt that even a little bit of vasculitis can play hell with the retinopathy). You have to be on guard for subtle signs that don't fit in with typical diabetes, like macular edema out of proportion to the microvascular damage, or excessive staining of the vessels and/or nerve on fluorescein angiogram. Recognizing the synergizing presence of uveitis is crucial because the addition of local steroids or systemic immunosuppression can really help control the retinopathy (Figure 1).

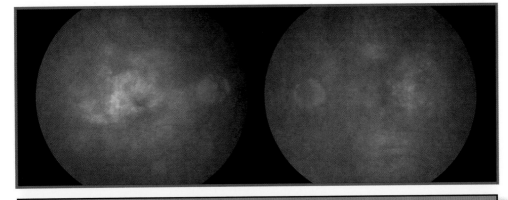

Figure 1. A patient with mild intermediate uveitis in the right eye and diabetic retinopathy alone in the left eye. Note the markedly asymmetrical macular edema. Also—and this is subtle—note the slightly increased disc staining, especially in the center of the nerve. These findings strongly suggest uveitis.

Some other examples of things that can rev up the retinopathy include hematologic problems such as anemias, lymphoproliferative disorders or dysproteinemias. If you are following someone for retinopathy and they suddenly have lots of new blot hemorrhages or mild vascular tortuosity, it is easy to think of the changes as just "worsening" retinopathy. If you had seen these patients de novo—without a history of diabetes—you would likely make the connection to a systemic hematologic disease much faster. Try to at least think about these things if a patient's fundus starts to look really bloody—and don't be afraid to check a CBC or serum protein electrophoresis like a real doctor.

Oh, and don't forget that if your patient is on Coumadin, they may have lots of creepy hemorrhages that suggest either hematologic or retinovascular problems, such as a central retinal vein occlusion. You can always check an INR if you are worried, but many times this is just something that goes along with diabetic retinopathy and Coumadin (kind of makes you wonder what their brains look like...).

And finally, never, never, never forget the usual suspects if the retinopathy is acting up with lots of hemorrhages, cotton wool spots and other background changes. These are: poor glucose control, accelerated hypertension, renal failure and hypercholesterolemia. This is a rehash of Chapters 5 and 20, but the message merits repetition. If you are sick of reading it, go find another textbook.

What if one eye is a lot worse than the other?

Keep in mind that something strange may be going on in a patient who has very asymmetric disease. Diabetic retinopathy is almost always asymmetric to some extent, but you should worry if there is a big difference between the two eyes. The uveitis patient shown above is one example of this.

However, there are two bad boys you *really* need to keep in mind: central retinal vein occlusion (CRVO) and ocular ischemic syndrome (OIS). Both of these can present with way more hemorrhages and more pronounced macular edema in the worse eye. Both entities can also cause venous dilation that can be quite subtle at first. Sometimes you have to study photos of each eye simultaneously to more easily identify the vascular changes that suggest one of these entities (Figure 2). If the worst eye also has anterior segment neovascularization, then it is practically screaming CRVO or OIS—make sure you listen. (Ocular ischemic syndrome is really bad for diabetics, and diabetics are more likely to get it because they are, well, diabetic. It is important enough that it gets its very own chunk of this chapter later on to help you sniff it out.)

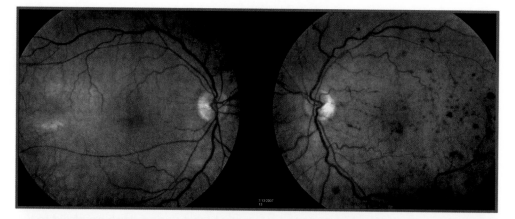

Figure 2. Asymmetric retinopathy due to a mild central retinal vein occlusion. Note the slightly dilated and tortuous veins, which suggest that the left eye has more going on than just accelerated background retinopathy.

If you think you are dealing with venous occlusive disease or ocular ischemia superimposed on diabetes, you have to deal with the ramifications of the diagnosis (e.g., check carotid Dopplers if you are worried about ischemia, consider a systemic work-up if you are worried about a vein occlusion and watch for anterior segment neovascularization for both). You also want to make darn sure the patient is aware of your concerns as you discuss the treatment and prognosis. He or she needs to know that everything you do may not work as well because of the double jeopardy and that the vision may worsen in spite of treatment and, in particular, how the eye may get neovascular glaucoma if the ischemia worsens.

(Remember Chapter 6 and the part about warning the patient that things may get worse, even with perfect treatment? Well, if your patient has diabetes and macular edema from a central retinal vein occlusion that you didn't recognize— and if that patient then gets neovascular glaucoma two weeks after you do the laser for edema—you *know* they will blame your focal for the nightmare they are about to experience. Not good.)*

---

* And they should blame you because you have screwed up twice:
    1. By missing the CRVO in the first place.
    2. If the macular edema was entirely due to a CRVO, it is a waste of time to do a laser—but that is a tale for different book.

Other thoughts on asymmetric disease:

As mentioned, diabetic retinopathy can be asymmetric just because it happens to be asymmetric. Sometimes this is handy because the first eye gives the patient a taste of what is in store for remaining eye if they don't take care of themselves. Do not hesitate to point this out to them if they don't realize it on their own.

In terms of disease pathology, though, there is one other issue that comes up occasionally in the literature: whether the asymmetric retinopathy is a manifestation of occult carotid disease. It has been suggested that a significant carotid obstruction can lower the blood pressure in the retinal vessels in the ipsilateral eye (unless there is collateral flow around the circle of Willis). The lower blood pressure turns out to be protective—the hydrostatic forces that eat away at blood vessels are lower—so the eye fed by the diseased carotid actually looks healthier.[2]

However, this effect is probably pretty rare, if it exists at all.[3] If carotid disease is going to cause a problem, it is much more likely to result in worsening of retinopathy from ischemia. The real question is whether you need to do carotid Dopplers on all patients with asymmetric disease. This is probably not necessary unless there is a big asymmetry that can't be explained by local eye conditions, or unless one eye develops anterior segment neovascularization. If you do Dopplers on everyone with just a bit of asymmetric disease, you may pick up something interesting on occasion, but it will probably have nothing to do with the retinopathy. Also, the patient may be more likely to end up at the vascular surgeon's office for no good reason. You decide…

Anyway, back to the differential diagnosis of diabetic retinopathy and the second scenario:

Things that can really make you look bad if they show up in a diabetic with no prior retinopathy and you think they are from diabetes.

The first section covered problems that can be "invisible" because they can superimpose themselves on pre-existing diabetic retinopathy, and you can miss them if you are not careful. Now it is time to turn to entities that, in and of themselves, can mimic diabetes. Most of these can be missed if they happen to show up in a diabetic patient—that is, you would be more likely to think of them if the patient wasn't diabetic. (Usually Occam's razor is spot-on, but sometimes it can slice you a piece of bad-diagnosis pie.)

Perhaps the most common troublemaker is a branch vein occlusion (BRVO). An acute BRVO can mimic diabetes if it is very mild, but usually the sectoral nature of the hemorrhages and the edema will tip you off. An old, chronic BRVO, however, can be a fooler because the vascular remodeling can spread across the horizontal midline, and the more acute findings that trigger the BRVO pattern-recognition algorithm in your head—like a localized sector of hemorrhage—are no longer present (Figure 3).

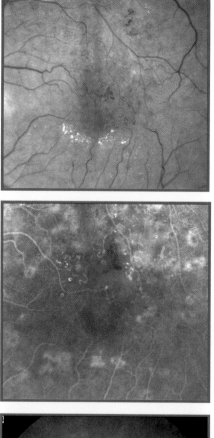

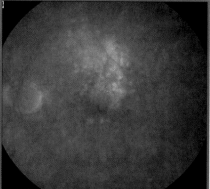

Figure 3. An old branch retinal occlusion simulating diabetic retinopathy. Note how the vascular changes can look much more like diabetes once the acute changes have resolved. In this case, there are also some hard exudates that have spread to the other side of the fovea, masking the fact that all the microvascular changes are localized above the fovea (something that would normally make you think of a BRVO). The early-phase angiogram clearly shows vascular remodeling in the distribution of a vein above the fovea and the late phase shows the leakage localized to the same area—this is where an angiogram can be very helpful to make the diagnosis. Note that the patient has already had grid laser to the area of leakage, including some grid spots below the fovea (suggesting that someone thought this was diabetes and added grid to non-pathologic retina).

Why is it important to make the distinction? One could argue that it isn't important, because you will still grid any swollen retina and you will still encourage the patient to take better care of their risk factors. However, this rationalization is not correct and can lead to big problems.

First of all, the late vascular remodeling that occurs with an old BRVO can simulate easily treatable microaneurysms. Usually these vascular changes are dilated vessels that may provide the only remaining circulation to the fovea. If you go after them like diabetic microaneurysms you could shut down the fovea. Bad move. BRVOs tend to need more of a grid thing rather than a "shoot red" thing. Plus, one does not tend to automatically treat macular edema from a BRVO in the same way one treats diabetic edema. (Usually the vision has to be 20/40 or worse to justify treatment, according to the Branch Vein Occlusion Study—grab a retina text for the full story on this.) Bottom line: If a patient has a local area of leakage that seems to respect the horizontal midline and does not have much in the way of vascular changes anywhere else, think BRVO and get an FA before you start cooking microaneurysms.

The second problem is that BRVOs can develop screwy-looking collateral vessels over time, and if you haven't realized you are dealing with a BRVO you can mistake them for proliferative disease. If you incorrectly do a PRP on such a patient you will be destroying retina needlessly—and until we figure out how to replace it you will be gaining some serious negative karma. To complicate matters, patients may develop true neovascularization secondary to a BRVO—and not just collateral vessels. These new vessels do need to be treated, but if you mistake them for proliferative diabetic retinopathy you will needlessly treat them with panretinal photocoagulation when they usually just need a sector of photocoagulation to treat the area of ischemia caused by the BRVO.

A central retinal vein occlusion can actually be a bit more problematic than a BRVO when it comes to distinguishing it from diabetic disease, and this is particularly true if the CRVO is mild. Because CRVOs are diffuse, rather than localized like a BRVO, they can simulate both new onset retinopathy or be hidden by preexisting retinopathy (see the prior section). It is a bit easier to sniff out a CRVO if there is no retinopathy to begin with because all the usual CRVO findings stand out as a sudden change and the unilaterality is telling.

> **You should keep in the very back of your mind** the possibility of bilateral mild CRVOs in a diabetic who suddenly develops retinopathy. If you have been following diabetics for a while, you know that they usually do not quickly go from zero retinopathy to lots of pathology. The new onset of bilateral disease with features that suggest a CRVO such as venous dilation and tortuosity should make you suspicious. Such a scenario is so unlikely that you will probably never see it, but bilateral CRVOs are almost always a sign of something bad and if you blow them off as diabetes you might miss life-threatening diseases.

Radiation retinopathy is another entity that can closely mimic diabetic retinopathy, but the history of radiation therapy will clue you in (Figure 4). Radiation retinopathy tends to be nastier than diabetes, especially in terms of capillary dropout and ischemia. It also tends to be more refractory to treatment than typical diabetes—and you and your patient need to know that the prognosis may not be as good if radiation damage is part of the problem. Where you need to be on your guard about this is with a known diabetic who didn't tell you—or whom you never asked—about prior radiation treatment. (Remember that stuff in medical school about PMH, ROS, PSH, etc.? This is where it does something more useful than allow you to bill a level-four visit.)

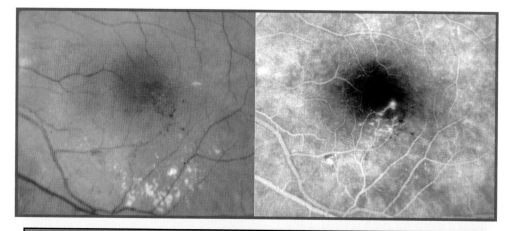

Figure 4. Radiation retinopathy. There is really nothing diagnostic about the appearance, although there is a sense that radiation creates more capillary dropout and ischemia than one would expect from a similar degree of diabetic retinopathy.

Idiopathic juxtafoveal telangiectasis type 2a (IJFT 2a) is another close mimic (Figure 5). There are several entities within the overall category of juxtafoveal telangiectases, but the type 2a subset is the most common and the one most likely to simulate diabetes. Plus, these patients are more likely to have diabetes—and if they aren't already diabetic, they are prone to becoming so. IJFT 2a is characterized by tiny microvascular abnormalities around the fovea, especially on the temporal side. The pathology tends to be very symmetrical. (If you think you have a unilateral case, you are most likely looking at an old, small BRVO with late vascular remodeling or, less likely, the type 1 subset of IJFT.[4]) The appearance on FA is also quite characteristic: There is a very symmetrical doughnut of leakage in the late phases, with more leakage on the temporal side of each fovea.

Texts often refer to the presence of "right-angle venules," a term that makes no sense unless you see a few of these patients. It refers to veins that drain the outer retinal capillaries. (The "right-angle" refers to the fact that, if you look closely, the tip of the venule seems to dive down—directly away from the observer—into the outer capillaries. It does *not* refer to a right-angle turn in the horizontal plane of the retina, which is what one might otherwise think.)

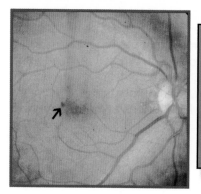

Figure 5-1. IJFT 2a. The microvascular changes are less obvious with a color photo, although there is a sense that the perifoveal veins are dilated. See Figure 5-4 for the FA, which is far more dramatic. There is a bit of pigment in the area of the abnormal vessels (arrow), which is not uncommon in this entity. Note the subtle grayish color to the perifoveal retina, which tends to be symmetrical—this suggests you are not dealing with diabetic disease.

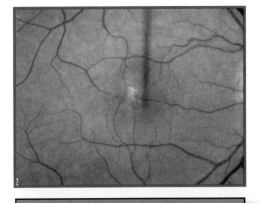

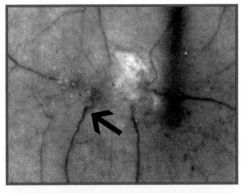

Figure 5-2. (Above) IJFT 2a. The dilated veins around the fovea are more obvious in a red free photo (different patient).

Figure 5-3. (Above) Close-up of Figure 5-2. The arrow shows a "right-angle vein." The view is not stereoscopic, but you can get a sense that the vein is diving down into the outer retina. You can also see some of the refractile deposits seen in IJFT 2a to the left of the fovea.

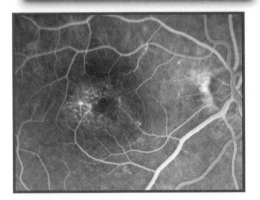

Figure 5-4. (Left) Early FA of IJFT 2a. You might call this diabetes, but note how the whole area around the fovea has an odd appearance and there are more abnormalities temporal to the fovea. There would also be a striking symmetry between the two eyes (see next figure).

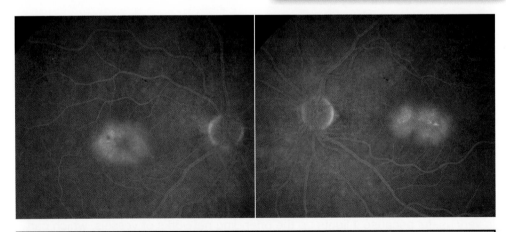

Figure 5-5. Late FA showing both eyes of a patient with IJFT 2a. Note the symmetric doughnut shape to the edema. If you do not think of this entity when you see this pattern, you may decide to use laser, which usually has no effect and can be counterproductive.

These patients can also get pigment clumping around the vascular abnormalities, as well as tiny golden refractile deposits near the fovea. Both findings are more prominent on the temporal side. OCT testing can show cystic changes, but there is usually a surprising lack of retinal thickening given the leakage seen on the angiogram.

Although patients tend to get gradual blurring of their vision over time, they do not get severe vision loss. However, a subset of patients can develop very unusual neovascular membranes within and beneath the retina, and these patients can lose a lot of vision if this process is not recognized.

It is very important to consider this entity because laser treatment will not work; in fact, it may make them worse. Repeat: It can make them worse. You should be embarrassed if you do consider lasering such patients, because it indicates you have switched off your brain and are going on pattern recognition alone: You are seeing the red spots and leakage on FA, but you are ignoring the fact that your brain and the OCT are telling you the retina is not very thick and both eyes are very symmetrical. Also, if the patient does get a neovascular membrane, they will then get definite retinal thickening. If you mistake this thickening for worsening diabetic edema, you will be encouraged to do more of the forbidden thing mentioned a few sentences ago. This will again have no useful effect and will now delay effective treatment, allowing your patient to get much worse.

If you think you do have a patient with IJFT 2a, you should congratulate yourself for making a relatively obscure diagnosis. However, there really is not much in the way of proven treatment for the leakage. People are always trying things, ranging from topical nonsteroidals to intravitreal therapy, so if you are considering the diagnosis it is best to get a retina consult to confirm it and to see what the treatment du jour may be.

The situation is quite different, though, if the patient does develop a neovascular membrane. There is a lot of data suggesting that anti-VEGF agents and/or photodynamic therapy with Visudyne may help prevent severe vision loss. Patients with this problem should be referred quickly and not allowed to languish in anyone's collection of patients with poor response to grid laser.

Another entity that can give you weird-looking vessels that may seem diabetic-ish at first is adult-onset Coats' disease. These patients have patches of irregular, bulb-like vessels that tend to leak much later in life relative to the eye-destroying type of Coats' disease that children get (in which the vessels are far more diffuse). This disease is strongly unilateral, and there are often far more hard exudates than one would see with typical diabetic retinopathy. An FA is very useful because it lights up the offending networks of vessels, which can look quite bizarre. It is important to distinguish this from regular diabetic disease because—unlike diabetic macular edema—you usually need to really treat these vessels aggressively in order to avoid letting the macula fill up with yellow fat.

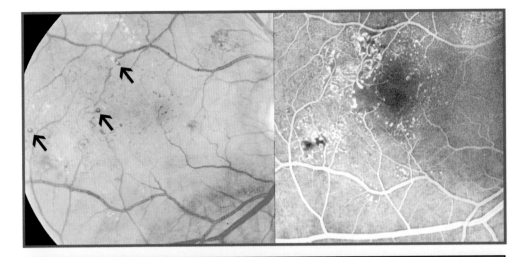

Figure 6. Adult-onset Coats' disease. (The color and the FA are from different points in time.) The arrows in the color photo show how the large, globular vessels will reflect the camera flash—showing up as a white dot on the red surface. The FA highlights the odd-looking bulbous vessels and the fact that the entire capillary bed is enlarged and irregular. This is very different from the more focal damage caused by diabetes. Finally, these photos are of early lesions. There will often be excessive amounts of hard exudates around the vascular lesions if the leakage is allowed to persist.

Most of the above entities have in common the fact that, at least at first, they mimic background diabetic changes. As mentioned at the beginning of the chapter, the differential is very different if you have a patient who is presenting with new vessels growing up off the retina. If you have a patient who presents with proliferative retinopathy and does turn out to have diabetes, and whose retinopathy is typical, you can relax and just follow the instructions in the rest of the book. (Well, relax only as far as making the diagnosis. Any patient who walks in the door with proliferative retinopathy is usually in big trouble, both from an ophthalmic standpoint and systemically.)

If the proliferative disease is atypical, then Table 1 can come in handy—as well as a textbook that covers all those diseases. There is, however, one proliferative disease in particular that you should keep in mind: proliferative retinopathy due to hemoglobin SC disease (especially if you have a patient population in the appropriate demographic). The far-peripheral nature of these vessels should make you think of this and prompt you to get a hemoglobin electrophoresis, even if the patient is diabetic. You do not want to mistake this entity for diabetes because treating SC disease requires a little more discretion—blasting away everything in the periphery is not necessarily a good thing for these patients. (Interestingly, the presence of hemoglobin SC does not seem to increase the risk of diabetic retinopathy.)[5]

But now on to the third scenario:

Patients *without* previously diagnosed diabetes and funny things in their retina that look diabetic.

This is usually the easiest because even an ophthalmologist can diagnose diabetes. (By the way, remember that we are talking about diagnosing Type 2 diabetes here—Type 1 does not show up in your clinic with retinopathy as a presenting sign. Those patients show up in the ER with polydipsia, polyuria and ketoacidosis.)

How do you diagnose diabetes? The pundits argue about this, but Table 3 shows the latest criteria. Just to make things confusing, there are three different sets of criteria: those from the European Diabetes Epidemiology Group, the American Diabetes Association and the World Health Organization. Fortunately, all are similar; the ADA criteria are used here.

There is increasing recognition that glucose intolerance is really more of a spectrum, rather than something that can be specified by a single number. This has led to the definition of prediabetic states such as "impaired glucose tolerance" or "impaired fasting glucose" (Table 4). Such patients are at risk for macrovascular disease, such as heart attack and stroke, and they represent a demographic with significant personal and public health consequences.

Table 3 / Criteria for the Diagnosis of Diabetes Mellitus

1. Symptoms of diabetes and a casual plasma glucose 200 mg/dl (11.1 mmol/l). Casual is defined as any time of day without regard to time since last meal. The classic symptoms of diabetes include polyuria, polydipsia, and unexplained weight loss.

or

2. Fasting plasma glucose 126 mg/dl (7.0 mmol/l). Fasting is defined as no caloric intake for at least 8 hours.

or

3. 2-hour plasma glucose 200mg/dl (11.1 mmol/l) during an oral glucose tolerance test. The test should be performed as described by the World Health Organization, using a glucose load containing the equivalent of 75 g anhydrous glucose dissolved in water. The oral glucose tolerance test is not recommended for routine clinical use.

(American Diabetes Association. Diabetes Care Vol 29 Supplement 1, 2006. Copyright 2006 The American Diabetes Association.)

Table 4 / Diagnostic Thresholds for Diabetes and
Lesser-Degrees of Impaired Glucose Regulation

Category	TEST	
	FPG	**2-h PG**
Normal	100 mg/dl (< 5.6 mmol/L)	<140 mg/dl (<7.8 mmol/L)
IFG	100 - 125 mg/dl (5.6-6.9 mmol/L)	-
IGT	-	140-199 mg/dl (7.8-11.0 mmol/L)
Diabetes*	≥126 mg/dl (≥7.0 mmol/L)	≥200 mg/dl (≥11.1 mmol/L)

IFG: Impaired Fasting Glucose
IGT: Impaired Glucose Tolerance
Note: IFG or IGT should be diagnosed only if diabetes is not diagnosed by the other test.
* The diagnosis of diabetes needs to be confirmed on a seperate day.

(Expert Committee on the Diagnosis and Classification of Diabetes Mellitus. Follow-up report on the diagnosis of diabetes mellitus. Diabetes Care 2003; 26:3160. Copyright 2003 The American Diabetes Association.)

Basically, the diagnosis of diabetes is established when a patient has a fasting blood glucose concentration of 126 mg/dL (7.0 mmol/L) or higher, or a random value of 200 mg/dL (11.1 mmol/L) or higher (confirmed by repeat testing). A hemoglobin A1c can also be helpful, although it is not yet felt to be a useful screening test until there is more standardization among various labs. If you think a patient has diabetes based on the eye, but the test results are equivocal, you can get more aggressive with a two-hour glucose tolerance test. This test is a hassle, though, and these patients should really be at their medical doctor getting the full systemic evaluation anyway. The point is that it should be fairly easy to rule in the diagnosis of diabetes if you are seeing worrisome changes in the fundus. Even if you don't diagnose frank diabetes, it is very likely the patient will turn out to have one of the prediabetic states (unless a completely different problem is causing their retinopathy). Note that it was once thought that "prediabetic" patients did not get microvascular changes in their retinas, but it is now recognized that such patients may have mild background findings, although they are unlikely to have any significant retinopathy.[6]

Oh yeah, there is one other simple thing to do if you have a patient with hemorrhages and swellings in the retina, and you may not think of it because you have been too busy memorizing how to talk to a patient about IOL reimbursement or something. You can look *extremely* bad, however, if you don't consider this particular entity and perform the simple test required to detect it. It was mentioned in Chapters 10, 20 and 22, and if you can't think of it, you really should go ahead and do that cornea fellowship. (Hint—look at Table 2).

If the patient has a few microvascular abnormalities but does not have any obvious systemic cause, recognize that recent population-based studies have found that perhaps 5 to 10% of patients over 40 to 50 years old can have occasional microaneurysms, retinal hemorrhages, and/or cotton wool spots. This may represent the effect of normal aging on the retinal vasculature, but it turns out that such patients are more likely to have problems such as hypertension or borderline glucose tolerance. Interestingly, these retinal findings can also be a marker for subclinical cerebrovascular and heart disease. In other words, if you have a patient with a few microaneurysms and no diabetes (and none of the other causes outlined in this chapter), don't just scratch your head and go "hrrrm." Inform their doctors and encourage these patients to get a complete physical, because the odds are good that something will turn up and finding it may improve their overall health.[7]

CHAPTER 26.1

Ocular Ischemic Syndrome — Thermonuclear Retinopathy

Global ocular ischemia may be very difficult to diagnose, particularly if the patient already has lots of diabetic eye disease. You won't see it very often unless you have a practice full of patients with awful disease, but you do not want to miss it if it does show up because it can be treatable if caught early and disastrous if caught late. In the past this syndrome has had a number of confusing names, including retinopathy of carotid insufficiency and venous stasis retinopathy (the latter being most problematic because some people have used the same term to describe a non-ischemic central retinal vein occlusion). Lately, everyone seems to agree that the most useful name is ocular ischemic syndrome (OIS), mostly because that is what the people at Wills Eye Hospital call it, and who's gonna argue with them?

Although OIS can be due to problems such as temporal arteritis or localized ophthalmic artery stenosis, by far the most common cause is atherosclerotic carotid artery obstruction. If it is related to carotid disease there is usually at least a 90% ipsilateral obstruction. Unfortunately, bilateral involvement is common, although it may be sequential. The thing about this entity is that it can show up in very sneaky ways, and you have to keep it in mind because about half of patients with OIS have co-existing diabetes.

Presentation

The actual presentation varies along a multifactorial grid that includes the amount of the obstruction, the rate of obstruction, and the nature of the intraocular response induced by the ischemia. And all of this is can be scrambled up if you are seeing it in the setting of diabetic retinopathy; early signs may be lost amongst the preexisting diabetic damage. This can be a problem. Remember the paragraph above that talked about the need to keep in mind the worst-case scenario when you make a given diagnosis? Well, OIS is usually one of those worst-case scenarios in the setting of aggressive diabetic retinopathy.

Almost all patients have some sort of visual symptoms. They may present with sudden vision loss if there is a relatively acute onset, although many times there is a gradual, variable amount of vision loss, often with episodes of amaurosis fugax that may be atypical. The symptoms can also seem non-specific, for instance, episodic blurring of vision or prolonged vision loss following exposure to bright lights. Patients may complain of colored vision, often reddish or violet in hue. Of course, some of these are the same symptoms that many diabetics routinely complain of once they have significant retinopathy—so you have to be listening for changes in the quality or degree of the complaints and whether they are unilateral. Patients may also complain of vague eyeaches, and a very characteristic symptom is a history of facial pain that improves with lying down.

The clinical findings can be quite varied in early, mild disease. Iris neovascularization is common, although it may be very subtle at first. Angle neovascularization leading to frank neovascular glaucoma is not far behind. However, one of the odd things about this entity is that the ischemic ciliary body may not be able to generate enough aqueous to elevate the pressure. Therefore, if the anterior segment neovascularization is subtle you may miss the diagnosis because there will be no elevated pressure to tip you off that something bad is happening. This is especially true if you are running a retina practice where patients are always seen after dilation—you won't see the new blood vessels and you won't have the pressure rise to make you suspicious.

By the way, the above problem means that if the patient ends up having carotid surgery, they may suddenly develop very high pressures as the ciliary body becomes perfused and starts to make aqueous. Both the patient and the vascular surgeon should be warned about this, and you should make arrangements to have someone else be on call to treat the miserable neovascular glaucoma that develops at 3:00 a.m. after their carotid is reopened.

> **There are some other presentations** that do need to be kept in mind to appreciate how peculiar this disease can be, even though they don't exactly intersect with the differential diagnosis of diabetes. OIS can result in corneal endothelial dysfunction with corneal edema and folds in Descemet's membrane. In an elderly patient with acute corneal decomposition, you have to think of OIS. OIS can also generate anterior uveitis with some anterior chamber cell and, rarely, even a keratic precipitate or two. Weird.

Posterior segment findings may be superficially similar to background diabetic retinopathy—and this is where you can easily miss the diagnosis. There may be retinal hemorrhages, but they tend to be further away from the posterior pole than typical diabetic hemorrhages, and they also tend to be larger and more blot-shaped (Figure 6). OIS, even without superimposed diabetes, can also cause neovascularization of the nerve, and there may even be microvascular changes such as capillary telangiectasis, microaneurysms, and macular edema.

Let's repeat one point here. OIS needs to be considered in a patient with unilateral cystic macular edema and not much diabetic retinopathy to explain it. (Assuming there are no other causes such as uveitis, an early CRVO, traction, etc.)

OIS patients will often have dilated veins, too, and the combination of the peripheral hemorrhages and venous changes may suggest a mild CRVO in addition to diabetes. Brown and Margargal [8] point out that in OIS, the veins may be dilated but not tortuous, which is different from a CRVO, in which the veins are usually both dilated and tortuous (Figures 7 and 8).

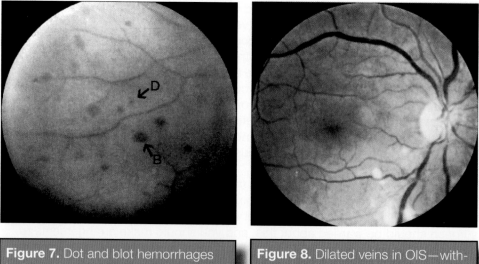

Figure 7. Dot and blot hemorrhages in the periphery of a patient with OIS. They are distributed more randomly and are "blotchier" than one would expect from diabetes. (Brown GC, Magargal LE. Int Ophthalmol 1988; 11:239-51.)

Figure 8. Dilated veins in OIS—without tortuosity. Also scattered cotton wool spots. (Sharma S, Brown GC, Ocular Ischemic Syndrome in Ryan SJ (ed.) Retina 4th Edition.)

Fluorescein angiography may be useful in sorting out the diagnosis. There is often a delay in both choroidal and retinal filling due to global ophthalmic artery hypoperfusion. There may also be late staining of the vessels and disc in early OIS, as well as the aforementioned macular edema. This may make one think of inflammatory disease, but the delayed circulation time should suggest OIS.

Digital ophthalmodynamometry is a classic physical exam maneuver that may allow you to make a very astute diagnosis of OIS, if you can actually remember to do it. Although there are devices to quantitate the pressure required to cause the central retinal artery to pulsate, it is easy to simply view the nerve and push on the eye with your finger. An eye with OIS will often show pulsations of the artery with only mild pressure (be sure you are not mistaking venous pulsations for arterial pulsations). Many times this finding is somewhat subtle and you need to compare one eye to the other to appreciate the difference. This does not necessarily make the diagnosis of OIS, but if it is present it really points you in the right direction.

Once you think you are dealing with OIS, the main concern is to make sure that there is no carotid disease that needs to be treated. The patient should have carotid Dopplers and be encouraged to get to their internist to make sure that they do not have any other vascular problems such as heart disease.

From an ophthalmic standpoint, if they develop neovascular glaucoma these patients usually need very aggressive panretinal photocoagulation, along with anti-VEGF therapy and whatever is needed to control the pressure. The PRP generally needs to be performed quickly and in high, painful doses, which tend to create symptomatic changes in vision. Patients really need to understand that you are fighting to save the eye—and they need to have appropriate expectations, because even if the treatment works these eyes don't tend to see well.

This discussion does not really do justice to this entity, and if you think you are dealing with OIS you should read some of the references that follow.[8-10] The main point is that this is a really bad thing to have happen to a diabetic eye, and it can be very subtle at first. However, you can help save both the patient's eye and their brain if you think about it.

References and Suggested Reading

1.   Jampol LM, Ebroon DA, Goldbaum MH. Peripheral proliferative retinopathies: an update on angiogenesis, etiologies and management. Surv Ophthalmol 1994;38:519-40.

2.   Basu A, Palmer H, Ryder RE, Taylor KG. Uncommon presentation of asymmetrical retinopathy in diabetes type 1. Acta Ophthalmol Scand 2004;82:321-3.

3.   Duker JS, Brown GC, Bosley TM, Colt CA, Reber R. Asymmetric proliferative diabetic retinopathy and carotid artery disease. Ophthalmology 1990;97:869-74.

4.   Sindt SJ, Oh K. Idiopathic juxtafoveal retinal telangiectasis: case report and literature review. Optometry 2001;72:228-33.

5.   Koduri PR, Patel AR, Bernstein HA. Concurrent sickle cell hemoglobin C disease and diabetes mellitus: no added risk of proliferative retinopathy? J Natl Med Assoc 1994;86:682-5.

6.   Tyrberg M, Melander A, Lovestam-Adrian M, Lindblad U. Retinopathy in subjects with impaired fasting glucose: the NANSY-Eye baseline report. Diabetes Obes Metab 2007.

7.   Wong TY, Klein R, Amirul Islam FM, et al. Three-year incidence and cumulative prevalence of retinopathy: the atherosclerosis risk in communities study. Am J Ophthalmol 2007;143:970-6.

8.   Brown GC, Magargal LE. The ocular ischemic syndrome. Clinical, fluorescein angiographic and carotid angiographic features. Int Ophthalmol 1988;11:239-51.

9.   Sivalingam A, Brown GC, Magargal LE. The ocular ischemic syndrome. III. Visual prognosis and the effect of treatment. Int Ophthalmol 1991;15:15-20.

10.   Sivalingam A, Brown GC, Magargal LE, Menduke H. The ocular ischemic syndrome. II. Mortality and systemic morbidity. Int Ophthalmol 1989;13:187-91.

Ryan SJ. Retina, 4th ed. Philadelphia: Elsevier Mosby, 2006. (Use this for further reading on a specific disease being considered in the differential diagnosis.)

McCulloch, DK. Diagnosis of Diabetes. UpToDate.com. May, 2008.

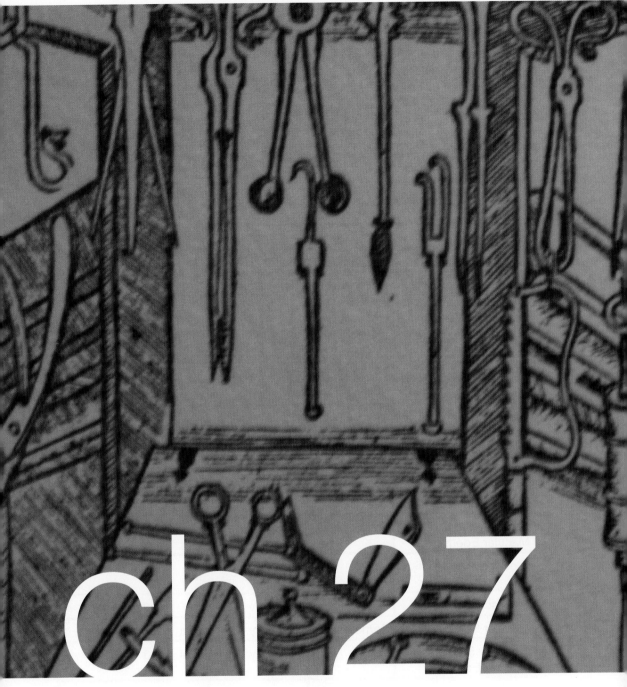

ch 27

Just How Often Do You Have to Drag Them Back, Anyway?

Table 1 is the best overview on how often one should follow up with and consider treating patients with different levels of retinopathy—it is based on the excellent review on diabetic retinopathy in the American Academy of Ophthalmology Focal Points series by Drs. Fong and Ferris.[1] It basically covers everything nicely.

Table 1 / Management of Diabetic Retinopathy

Level of Retinopathy	Focal Laser	Scatter Laser (PRP)	Follow-Up Interval (months)
Mild NPDR			
No Macular Edema	No	No	12
Macular Edema	No	No	4-6
Clinically Significant Macular Edema	Yes	No	2-4
Moderate NPDR			
No Macular Edema	No	No	6-8
Macular Edema	No	No	4-6
Clinically Significant Macular Edema	Yes	No	2-4
Severe NPDR			
No Macular Edema	No	Consider	3-4
Macular Edema	Sometimes	Consider After Focal	2-3
Clinically Significant Macular Edema	Yes	Consider After Focal	2-3
Proliferative Diabetic Retinopathy			
No Macular Edema	No	Probably	2-3
Macular Edema	Sometimes	Probably After Focal	2-3
Clinically Significant Macular Edema	Yes	Probably After Focal	2-3
High-Risk PDR			
No Macular Edema	No	Yes	2-3
Macular Edema	Usually	Yes	1-2
CSME	Yes	Yes	1-2

(Reproduced, with permission, from Fong DS, Ferris FL, Focal Points: Clinical Modules for Ophthalmologists, "Practical Management of Diabetic Retinopathy," American Academy of Ophthalmology, 2003.)

However, some patients do not quite fit into a table, so here are some other things to consider:

First of all, there is some controversy about how often diabetics should be screened if they have no retinopathy. For instance, there is good evidence that suggests that older Type 2 diabetics can be screened every two years until they begin to develop retinopathy.[2] Also, for some reason retinopathy is vanishingly rare before the onset of puberty. As a result, the American Diabetes Association has a more complicated recommendation for pre-pubertal patients with Type 1 diabetes: They should have their first screening examination within three to five years after the diagnosis of diabetes once the patient is age 10 years or older.

Rather than trying to figure out what the preceding sentence means, or trying to remember which older patients are due for their bi-annual examination, it seems much simpler to just insist that all diabetics get examined once a year. Diabetics are understandably not enthusiastic about screening examinations, and human nature is human nature. (How often do you see your dentist?) It is all too easy for patients to neglect screening examinations, especially if they are asymptomatic. Then, after a few years go by and they begin to have symptoms from advanced disease, they suddenly remember to get an exam—but it may be too late. It makes sense to have diabetics of all types and ages get used to the idea that an annual eye exam is just part of their life.

The counter-argument is that annual examinations increase overall healthcare costs. It would certainly be great to spread out the examinations if everyone lived in a perfect world where every patient could be tracked perfectly. However, in the world where most of us live it is better to train them to have an annual eye exam than to spread out the visits and risk losing them to follow up—an eventuality that could end up costing everyone a lot more.

> **Please note** that the preceding discussion refers to patients who are known to have diabetes and are known to have no retinopathy. Any older patient with newly diagnosed diabetes absolutely needs an examination at the time of diagnosis. Period. There is a significant chance that they may have smoldering retinopathy due to long-standing undiagnosed diabetes, and an eye exam is at the top of their list of things to do.

There are also some other factors to consider when deciding how often to monitor patients once they do have some degree of retinopathy. An extremely important factor is the rate of disease progression. For instance, a patient who quickly goes from minimal background retinopathy to more advanced disease is very worrisome and should be monitored more frequently than the table may suggest. On the other hand, a patient with old, treated proliferative retinopathy that has been stable for years may only need one or two exams per year. Another factor usually related to progression is—once again—the patient's degree of systemic control. A poorly controlled patient is always at higher risk for getting into trouble (and at higher risk for being lost to follow up), and should be kept on a tighter leash in terms of return-visit frequency.

An additional factor is whether you are seeing the patient for the first time. Unless you have their old records, you have no way of knowing whether such patients have progressive disease. There is nothing wrong with bringing a patient back sooner than their degree of retinopathy would suggest in order to be sure that they are stable. You can reassure yourself about the rate of a patient's progression and reinforce the need to follow up—two for one!

Also, remember the effect that pregnancy can have on diabetic retinopathy. Refer to Chapter 22 for the suggested examination schedule for that particular situation—especially the part about encouraging diabetic women to have an eye exam well before they even *think* about getting pregnant.

Finally, recall the caveats about financial concerns mentioned in Chapter 21. Patients without insurance may simply be unable to afford returning for routine exams, and you should make sure that they are welcome regardless of their ability to pay. It is a lot easier—and just plain nicer—to do a quick diabetic screening exam for free than to make the patient and society pay for livelong disability resulting from preventable vision loss.

References

1.   Fong DS, Ferris FL. Practical Management of Diabetic Retinopathy. American Academy of Ophthalmology Focal Points 2003;21.
2.   Kristinsson JK. Diabetic retinopathy. Screening and prevention of blindness. A doctoral thesis. Acta Ophthalmol Scand Suppl 1997:1-76.

APPENDIX
Infrared Techniques

Infrared diode lasers are cheaper yet durable because they are a simpler design. For this reason they may be the laser of choice in situations where financial resources are limited or if the laser can't be pampered and babied like in your nice cushy clinic. There is also data that suggests infrared treatment is as effective as green for diabetic retinopathy, although there are nowhere near as many patients in these studies as in the DRS and ETDRS.[1-3] However, you can't just sit down at an infrared laser and assume you can treat with the same techniques you would use for a green laser. This would be a Very Bad Thing.

Infrared is much trickier to use because the burns can seem unpredictable. They are, in fact, predictable, but it just plain takes a lot of experience and you really need to be aware of the degree of pigment in both the choroid and retinal pigment epithelium as you treat. Green light hits the RPE like a hammer hitting a nail—all the heat you would ever need for a burn is right there. Infrared is not as well absorbed by the RPE and penetrates deeper, so you actually need to heat up both the RPE and inner choroid to get a burn. Don't be surprised if you need to use two to three times more power to do an infrared treatment compared to the powers you would use with a green laser. If there is not much pigment you need to really crank up the power—sometimes it is impossible to get a burn in very pale fundi with an infrared laser.

> Although using an infrared laser can be difficult at first, it does come in handy when the view is hazy. Recall that shorter wavelengths are scattered more than longer wavelengths and that infrared is less absorbed by just about everything in the eye (refer back to Figure 1 in Chapter 3). All of this means that it can get through media opacities much better than visible wavelengths.

Also, the way an infrared burn develops is different from that of a burn using a green laser. With a green laser, the burn intensity gradually increases as you increase the power; there is a nice, gentle linear relationship that has room for error. The retinal response to infrared is more like an "S"-shaped curve, with the steep part starting just when you can see a burn. In other words, a small increase in the power can have a big effect on how hot your burn is once you start getting some uptake.

At first, the infrared burn tends to be elusive; you will see nothing and you will keep turning the power up and up—which can be a creepy feeling. Then, once you start to see some early graying, you have to be very careful because even a tiny increase in power can dramatically increase the intensity of the burn.

This also means that the laser-tissue interaction is much less forgiving. For instance, if you have found a good power, you still have to be very vigilant about the level of pigmentation at the site of treatment. If you move into an area of darker pigmentation you can blow things apart suddenly and unexpectedly—especially if you have fallen into "green-laser mode" and are mechanically stomping away on the foot pedal without paying close attention.

Another difference between green and infrared is that the desired end point for a burn is much milder than with a green laser. A grayish-white or whitish burn that might be OK with green will be quite hot with infrared, and you will be treating at the limit of safety. Usually a light graying will do the trick—you can get nasty scars, more pain and maybe even a choroidal hemorrhage if you try to create burns similar to those you would expect with a green laser. Less is definitely more with infrared.

The infrared is also far more demanding of the quality of your focus. Even a slight astigmatic oval or a slight defocusing in the anterior-posterior direction will totally block your ability to create a burn. Conversely, if you choose your power using a spot that is a little out of focus, you can cause a bad burn if you suddenly snap into accurate focus as you are working.

All of this means time and patience. In the beginning you may feel that each spot is taking hours as you fuss with the power and duration settings, and there is no question that each spot does require a lot more finesse. This can be very tedious if you are trying to do a fast and furious PRP, but with experience this becomes much less of a problem.

Perhaps the best way to use an infrared is to use your foot to adjust the power. In other words, pick a duration that is 50 to 100% longer than you might use for green (say .3 second if you normally use .15 for green). Then get the power up to where you are getting the burn you want in lighter areas—remember this may be two to three times the power you would use for green. (Note: You may have to turn the aiming beam way down to be able to watch how the tissue responds to the laser as you apply the power. If the aiming beam is bright, you cannot see subtle changes in the tissue underneath it.)

Once you have a good setting that is giving you reasonable burns, you can then carefully move to more pigmented areas and be prepared to pull your foot off the pedal as soon as you see a burn begin. This way you do not need to be constantly adjusting the power up and down depending on the pigmentation—you can simply change how long you keep the pedal to the metal for each burn. This approach is still fussy, but less time-intensive than resetting the power every five burns or so (which is what will happen with infrared if you are keeping your foot down for the entire duration of every pulse). This technique was discussed in Chapter 9—the difference is that the technique is a luxury with the green but it is more of a necessity with infrared. (Chapter 9 also talked about defocusing the spot to help you control the energy density without having to keep adjusting the laser controls. You can try this with infrared, but usually this wavelength is merciless when it comes to proper focus, so this trick is not as useful as with green.)

There is one other problem with infrared: Because the burns tend to be deeper, patients tend to feel them much more. You can try the usual things—shorter duration, smaller spot, etc., but many times you can't change these settings too much without diminishing your ability to control the safety of the burn. You may need to use more retrobulbar anesthesia than you would with a green laser. If you bought an infrared to save money and you are in the middle of a big city in a developed country, you will have a problem because patients may drift away to other docs with polite green lasers. If you are in the middle of nowhere and using infrared, then your audience is more captive—so just try to go slow and be as gentle as possible. (On the other hand, many patients prefer the infrared because there is no visible flash of light and they feel the treatment is therefore less intense.)

The infrared laser is not something you should start your laser career with, if at all possible; it is much easier to learn treatment techniques with a green laser. If you must dive in with infrared, try to do a bunch of PRPs first so that you can get a good sense of how this wavelength behaves before you start treating the macula. This is because you can get nasty burns really fast if you are not careful—something that is not a good idea around the fovea. Also, you usually cannot get microaneurysms to change color with infrared, so don't go crazy turning up the power and trying to whiten microaneurysms.

If you are treating macular edema with infrared, it is much better get in a *very* light grid of burns and then wait and see how the patient does. You can do focal treatment as well, but definitely don't try for a color change. Instead, just include the focal treatment as part of the grid. You can always add more treatment over time if necessary—don't wallpaper the macula with a lot of whitish infrared burns because you will leave a very destructive legacy.

> **One thing to keep in mind** is that if you are using an infrared laser made by Iridex, you may have the capability of doing micropulse laser. (See Chapter 3 for a brief description and references.) Your laser representative can help you determine whether this is a possibility. Many of these lasers were purchased with no intention of using the micropulse settings and the original owner may not even know whether this is an option.
>
> Micropulsing an infrared laser is one technique for creating subthreshold burns, i.e., burns that you cannot detect visually. It is felt that such burns may have a physiologic effect without causing much damage. There are no large controlled trials that prove the efficacy of these approaches, but it is worth watching the literature on all these techniques, because in the future the goal may be to treat edema with "low-impact" laser combined with pharmaceutical interventions. The fact that you are reading this appendix suggests that you may be well positioned to take advantage of these techniques if they are proven effective.

Please note that this section is just a brief introduction to the art of lasering in the infrared. If you are learning your trade on this type of laser, hopefully you have a kindly instructor who will take the time to nurture your skills personally. Infrared can be a great wavelength because it can penetrate media opacities and it can be much more affordable, especially in developing countries. It is just that it is a tricky thing to master, so take your time, be careful with your settings, stay very attuned to the amount of pigment in the tissue you are treating and pay close attention to your focus.

References

1.   Akduman L, Olk RJ. Diode laser (810 nm) versus argon green (514 nm) modified grid photocoagulation for diffuse diabetic macular edema. Ophthalmology 1997;104:1433-41.
2.   Bandello F, Brancato R, Trabucchi G, Lattanzio R, Malegori A. Diode versus argon-green laser panretinal photocoagulation in proliferative diabetic retinopathy: a randomized study in 44 eyes with a long follow-up time. Graefes Arch Clin Exp Ophthalmol 1993;231:491-4.
3.   Ulbig MW, Hamilton AM. [Comparative use of diode and argon laser for panretinal photocoagulation in diabetic retinopathy]. Ophthalmology 1993;90:457-62.

INDEX